THERAPEUTIC INTERVENTIONS FOR PARENT-CHILD CONTACT ISSUES

THERAPEUTIC INTERVENTIONS FOR PARENT-CHILD CONTACT ISSUES

A Clinician's Guide

By

KELLEY BAKER, PHD

and

AMY EICHLER, PHD

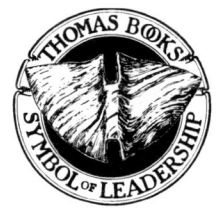

CHARLES C THOMAS, PUBLISHER, LTD.
Springfield, Illinois • USA

Published and Distributed Throughout the World by

CHARLES C THOMAS • PUBLISHER, LTD.
2600 South First Street
Springfield, Illinois 62704

This book is protected by copyright. No part of
it may be reproduced in any manner without written
permission from the publisher. All rights reserved.

© 2025 by CHARLES C THOMAS • PUBLISHER, LTD.

ISBN 978-0-398-09461-4 (paper)
ISBN 978-0-398-09462-1 (ebook)

Library of Congress Catalog Card Number: 2024052035 (print)
2024052036 (ebook)

With THOMAS BOOKS *careful attention is given to all details of manufacturing and design. It is the Publisher's desire to present books that are satisfactory as to their physical qualities and artistic possibilities and appropriate for their particular use.* THOMAS BOOKS *will be true to those laws of quality that assure a good name and good will.*

Printed in the United States of America
MX-C-1

Library of Congress Cataloging-in-Publication Data

Names: Baker, Kelley (Psychologist), author. | Eichler, Amy, author.
Title: Therapeutic interventions for parent-child contact issues : a
   clinician's guide / by Kelley Baker, PhD and Amy Eichler, PhD
Description: Springfield, Illinois : Charles C Thomas, Publisher, Ltd.,
   [2025] | Includes bibliographical references and index.
Identifiers: LCCN 2024052035 (print) | LCCN 2024052036 (ebook) | ISBN
   9780398094614 (paperback) | ISBN 9780398094621 (ebook)
Subjects: LCSH: Parental alienation syndrome. | Children of divorced
   parents--Mental health. | Custody of children--Psychological aspects.
Classification: LCC RJ506.P27 B35 2025 (print) | LCC RJ506.P27 (ebook) |
   DDC 618.92/89--dc23/eng/20241228
LC record available at https://lccn.loc.gov/2024052035
LC ebook record available at https://lccn.loc.gov/2024052036

This book is dedicated to all the many social scientists and clinicians who helped us find our way by their willingness to share their knowledge, share their time, endure the attacks of media and unhealthy parents, and publish their knowledge.
Thank you.

Rebecca Bailey	*Janet Johnson*
Amy J. L. Baker	*Demosthenes Lorandos*
Nicholas Bala	*Steve Miller*
William Bernet	*Diedra Rand*
Michael Bone	*Randy Rand*
Bill Eddy	*Katheen Reay*
Robert Evans	*Richard Sauber*
Barbara Fidler	*Lynn Steinberg*
Steven Friedlander	*Judith Wallerstein*
Richard Gardner	*Marjorie Walters*
Linda Gottlieb	*Richard Warshak*
Jonathan Gould	*Karen Woodall*
Joan Kelly	*Nick Woodall*
Jennifer Harman	

INTRODUCTION

This book is for clinicians – therapists, counselors, clinical social workers, and psychologists, who work directly with clients going through separation and divorce. While the information gained in most graduate programs and internships prepares the clinician for working with unhealthy family dynamics, it does not prepare practitioners for the unique demands of working with families in custody litigation. Family court judges need skilled mental health professionals to assess and treat families in divorce.

Judges and lawyers are not mental health experts. They rely on the input of psychological experts to make decisions to help the children and parents in their courtrooms. For the mental health professional interested in such work, the personal and professional rewards can be great, but the emotional and professional costs can be high if you do not educate yourself fully before attempting this type of work.

The authors are licensed clinicians who stepped (or fell) into working with this special population, unknowingly entering a kind of work that was not supported by their years of training acquired during graduate school. The theories and techniques that proved helpful were found from social science research and practitioners who were attempting to work with and understand this population. As such, many of the ideas and suggestions in this book can be attributed to researchers and clinicians who were exploring and writing about an emerging area of science. Their work provided the authors with guidance, suggestions, techniques, and resources when clients were demonstrating behaviors that did not fit the theories we learned in school and practicum. As such, the treatment approaches offered in this book are grounded in social science research and supported by existing peer-reviewed literature, or they have practical value from the authors' experience.

Chapters are presented in a consistent format similar to training seminars and manuals. They begin with learning objectives and, when appropriate, end with a summary of suggested resources labeled as "Clinician's Toolbox." The resources include forms, supplies, media, and other practical reminders a therapist might consider adding to their repertoire of techniques when working with this population. Case vignettes provide real-life examples taken from the authors' professional experience. The identifying information has been altered to protect confidentiality.

The book begins with a brief historical look at divorce and custodial issues to provide the reader with a basic understanding of how high-conflict divorce came to be a more common issue seen in therapy offices across the globe. Divorce is not a new phenomenon for families. Practitioners have been helping this population for years. However, high-conflict divorce presents challenges for the therapist that are unique from the average, moderately acrimonious divorce experience.

The next two chapters discuss the causes for high- conflict dynamics and assessment procedures appropriate for private practitioners. There are various family dynamics, mental health disorders, and legal agendas that exacerbate conflict during separation and divorce. Some of these dynamics may begin before the separation occurs. Children are often caught in the middle of warring parents, and the results can be devastating to the parent-child relationships and future development. High-conflict divorce litigation can last for the entirety of the child's developmental years. Clinicians can only address this unique experience by identifying the causal factors and their impact on development.

Chapter 3 discusses assessment procedures appropriate for clinicians providing therapeutic services. Treatment planning is based on accurate assessment, but the information available to the clinician may be limited unless there is a forensic evaluation available to review. The separation and divorce specialist approaches intake differently than the therapist working with other populations.

Chapter 4 focuses on cases involving abuse allegations. It provides suggestions for obtaining critical information, orients clinicians to the components used to differentiate justified and unjustified reasons for contact refusal, and makes suggestions for treatment while forensic investigators assess allegations. Understanding a child's resistance to a parent during separation and divorce can be complicated when the parents have contradicting views of what is causing the child's resistance. This is a common occurrence in high-conflict divorce and poses particular challenges to the private practitioner who is not conducting a forensic evaluation but needs to understand the causes for the resistance.

When current or potential litigation lurks in the background, clinicians should proceed with healthy skepticism and cautious optimism. This approach is not taught in most graduate programs across the country because training assumes that the average private practice is built on clientele who want to be there, have complete confidentiality to discuss their deepest conflicts, and have a genuine agenda of self-improvement.

Chapter 5 discusses the terminology and diagnostic codes clinicians should use when working with children affected by loyalty binds and unhealthy parental alignments. Agreement on the "best" terminology continues to be debated by leaders in the field. However, the authors provide the most widely accepted terminology, so the reader is equipped with the vocabulary to clearly describe and understand case details (Bernet et al., 2021). The legal field has terminology to describe professionals with special skills and who play specific roles within the family court system. Mental health professionals working with this population need to understand the definitions and responsibilities of these roles in case they are asked to fulfill the role or if they are required to interface with someone else appointed in that role.

The DSM provides specific diagnostic codes applicable to clients involved in a contentious divorce situation. The accurate diagnosis of the client's experience in the family may be accompanied by other disorders commonly used in therapeutic practice (i.e., mood, anxiety, behavioral, and personality disorders). However, the section of the DSM on relational issues includes diagnoses that were specifically meant to address family conflict during separation and divorce and the unique experiences possible in that situation (APA, 2013). An expanded discussion of the diagnostic definitions is included in this chapter.

Chapters 6 through 10 are treatment chapters and provide clinicians with treatment goals and common techniques used to reach those goals. Chapter 6 speaks to the overall process of treatment planning. Chapter 7 focuses on therapy with a child who may be caught in the middle of parents fighting over custody or struggling with normal grief and loss and adjustment issues. Clinicians are in a unique position to provide a psychologically safe space for children to process complex emotions related to divorce and parental conflict.

Chapter 8 provides guidance on treatment and techniques when therapists are working with a parent who is strongly aligned with a child. Many parents do not understand the detrimental effect their behaviors have on their children, but once they understand how they may be harming their children, many will change course, and damage to the children can be avoided. Also discussed in this chapter is how some parents will not change their negative behaviors despite education and are willing to psychologically abuse their children to maintain control and exclude the other parent. This group of parents requires the most resources to manage and can cause immense damage to their children. Mental health professionals are often targets for exploitation and manipulation by these parents (Warshak, 2020). Suggestions for dealing with this type of parent and knowing when to terminate services are provided.

Chapter 9 addresses the unique needs of a parent who has been rejected by their child or whose child is showing resistance towards them during separation and divorce. Resistance can be the result of many different things, but the loss of a child adds another layer to the emotional and psychological issues related to divorce. These parents are some of the most vulnerable and heartbroken. They are at a higher risk of suicide (Harman et al., 2022) and sometimes behave irrationally, which pushes the children further away and complicates the custody issues (Johnston et al., 2001).

Chapter 10 is designed for the clinician working with all the family members in family therapy. While the treatment approach for individual members may include some of the suggestions in the previous chapters, family therapy provides unique opportunities to address unhealthy alignments and family dynamics that create conflict. Many of the dynamics are entrenched and developed long before the separation occurred. Familiar dynamics such as triangulation are discussed. Techniques and resources for dealing with reunification issues are provided for the family therapist treating resistance and refusal issues between a child and a parent.

Chapter 11 describes specialized interventions used for severe cases of parental alienation. This chapter also discusses treatment team models for managing interventions requiring multiple mental health professionals. In many cases, one very strong family therapist is more successful in helping to stabilize a family in divorce than a larger team consisting of several individual therapists for reasons discussed in the chapter (Walters & Friedlander, 2016). The role of a treatment team lead is described, including the experience needed in this role and their duties. The benefits of a treatment team lead are discussed.

The book closes with a chapter on how mental health professionals working with this population can protect themselves from aggressive lawyers, mentally ill clients, and licensing complaints. The authors provide treatment suggestions and tools in this book that are supported by science, which is the best form of protection and ensures that the services provided are most likely to relieve pain and stabilize the family. Over the years, the authors have identified other ways to ensure protection by requesting specific wording in court orders, maintaining adequate notes that are helpful but also protective of the client, and maintaining adequate communication with clients while also maintaining firm boundaries, all of which are included in this chapter.

We hope you find the information and resources in this book helpful as you navigate providing services to families in divorce. It is not easy work and not meant for everyone. It requires a mental health professional who can contain the depth of the family's emotional pain, even when it manifests as attacks on the professionals trying to help. Working in this area requires bravery and resilience as you interact with vulnerable, fearful parents and aggressive lawyers. Clinicians will need to develop a self-care routine to maintain their own emotional health and guard against burnout. Our goal is to prepare you for the needs of this population and arm you with the information necessary to help families and protect yourself.

CONTENTS

                                                                       Page

Introduction vii

Chapter 1. A BRIEF HISTORY OF DIVORCE AND PARENT-CHILD CONTACT ISSUES 3
    History of Child Custody 3
    History of Parent-Child Contact Issues 6
        Severe Contact Refusal 8
        Parental Alienation 8

Chapter 2. CAUSES OF PARENT-CHILD CONTACT ISSUES 15
        Loyalty Conflicts 16
        Reactions to Circumstances of Divorce 17
        Parental Conflict Pre- and Post Separation 18
            Intimate Partner Violence/Domestic Violence ... 18
        Parent Characteristics 20
        Attachment 22
        Child Characteristics 23
            Age/Developmental Preferences 23
            Vulnerability/Resilience 25
            Stubborn Child 25
            Anxiety or Depression 26
    Family Dynamics 26
        Unhealthy Alignments 26
            Triangulation 26
            Enmeshment 27
            Parental Alienation 28
            Estrangement 30
            Parental Alienation/Estrangement- Hybrid Case ... 31
            Family of Origin Issues 33

Chapter 3. ASSESSMENT PROCEDURES FOR MENTAL HEALTH
PROFESSIONALS (CLINICIANS) 34
    Assessment Resources for Clinicians 35
        Pertinent Legal Information 35
        Collateral Consults 37
        Testing Instruments 38
        Historical Timelines 40
        Family of Origin Information 40
        Transitions and Exchanges 41
        Signs of Contact Issues in the Therapy Room 42
            Child as a Client 42
            Parents as Clients 43
        Reactions to Intervention 44
        Neutrality Bias 46
        Areas of Investigation for Causes of Resistance 48

Chapter 4. CASES INVOLVING ABUSE ALLEGATIONS:
DIFFERENTIATING BETWEEN ESTRANGEMENT AND PARENTAL
ALIENATION 52
    The Five-Factor Model of Parental Alienation 57
        Factor One 58
        Factor Two 59
        Factor Three 60
        Factor Four 63
        Factor Five 67

Chapter 5. DIAGNOSTIC CONSIDERATIONS 71
        Child Affected by Parental Relationship Distress
        (CAPRD) 72
        Parent-Child Relational Problem (PCRP) and Child
        Psychological Abuse 74
        Interpersonal Violence and Distress 75
    Parental Alienation 76
        Levels of Resistance and Alienating Behaviors 77
            Mild Symptoms of PA 77
            Moderate Symptoms of PA 78
            Severe Symptoms of PA 79

Chapter 6. TREATMENT PLANNING 80
    Rapport Building 81
        Assessing Motivation 81
        Legal Orders 82
        Intake Process 83
    Forms of Resistance 83
        Scheduling Issues 84
        Extracurricular Activities 86
        Stalling the Start of Therapy 86
        Intrusiveness 87
        Child's Resistance to Therapy 88
    Why Traditional Therapy May Not Work 89
        Assessment 91
        Treatment Planning 93
        Formalized Treatment Agreements 94

Chapter 7. TREATMENT WITH THE CHILD 97
    Therapeutic Foci of Treatment 99
        Lifting the Burden 99
        Providing Protected Psychological Space 101
        Finding Authentic Experience 102
        Mild, Moderate, or Severe 102
    Goals and Techniques of Treatment 103
        Goal #1 Build Rapport 103
            Empathy 104
            Building a Covert Therapeutic Alliance 105
        Goal #2-Build Self-Esteem 106
            Techniques 108
        Goal #3-Help Child Individuate from Both Parents ... 108
            Techniques 109
        Goal #4-Develop Critical Thinking skills 112
            Techniques 113
        Goal #5-Integrate Psychological Split 117
            Techniques 118
        Goal #6-Decrease Anxiety and Trauma Responses 118
            Techniques 118
        Goal #7-Decrease Shame and Guilt 120
    Psychological Instruments 121
    Recommendations When Progress Stalls 122

Chapter 8. TREATMENT WITH THE FAVORED PARENT 125
   Therapeutic Foci of Treatment 125
   Goals and Techniques 126
      Goal #1-Follow the Court Order 127
      Goal #2-Understand Their Own Family of Origin
      Dynamics 127
      Goal #3-Support the Relationship Between the Child
      and the Targeted Parent 128
      Goal #4-Increase Insight and Take Responsibility 130
         Cognitive Distortions 130
         Parental Alienation Strategies 131
         Suggestibility and False Memories 133
      Goal #5-Increase Ability to Cooperatively
      Parallel Parent 133
   Mental Health Issues that May Limit Progress 135
   Recommendations When Progress Stalls 137

Chapter 9. TREATMENT WITH THE TARGETED PARENT 141
   Therapeutic Foci of Treatment 141
   Goals and Treatment 142
      Goal #1-Build Rapport and Trust 142
         Acknowledging Their Unique Experience 142
         Getting to Know the Child 144
      Goal #2-Shift From Anger and Betrayal to Empathy
      and Compassion 145
      Goal #3-Improve Parenting Skills 147
         Parenting and Parental Conflict 147
      Parenting Alienated Children 147
         Developmentally Appropriate Parenting 148
         Preparing for Reunification 149
      Goal #4-Increase Feelings of Hope and Empowerment .. 150
      Goal #5-Coping with Grief and Loss 156
         Ambiguous Loss 157
         Increasing Support 158
         Processing Ambiguous Loss 158
      Goal #6-Preparing the Parent for Therapeutic
      Contact with the Child 168

    Goal #7-Preparing the Parent to Receive the Child in
    Their Home 169
      Safety Plans 169
      Diffusing Conflict... 170
   Conclusion 170

Chapter 10. TREATMENT WITH THE FAMILY 172
   Therapeutic Foci of Treatment....................................... 174
   Goals and Techniques.. 175
    Working with the Parents... 175
     Goal #1-Establish Expectations for the
     Therapeutic Process 176
     Goal #2-Establish Healthy Communication
     Between the Parents 176
     Goal #3-Establish Healthy Boundaries Between
     Households.. 176
    Parent and Family Member Pledge to Child................ 177
    Working with Favored Parent-Child Dyad.................... 178
     Goal #1-Establish Healthy Boundaries Between
     Households.. 178
     Goal #2-Favored Parent to Support the
     Relationship Between Child and Target
     Parent.. 180
    Working with the Target Parent-Child Dyad................ 182
     Goal #1-Restore the Authority of the Target
     Parent.. 183
     Goal #2-Address Real Relationship Obstacles .. 184
     Goal #3-Correctively Re-Experience the Family .. 185
    Considerations with Siblings.. 187
   Recommendations When Progress Stalls 188

**Chapter 11. TREATMENT TEAM MODELS OF INTERVENTION
FOR SEVERE CASES OF PARENTAL ALIENATION** 190
   Family Bridges 191
   Turning Points for Families.. 194
   The Family Reflections Reunification Program (FRRP).. 195
   Therapeutic Treatment Teams 197

Chapter 12. PROFESSIONAL LIABILITY AND PROTECTING
YOURSELF 205
        Social Media 207
        Continuing Education 207
        Review Treatment Progress 208
        Court-Ordered Therapy 210
        Professional Role Boundaries 213
        Assessing Treatment Effectiveness 214
        Testifying in Court 215

Subject Index 237

THERAPEUTIC INTERVENTIONS FOR PARENT-CHILD CONTACT ISSUES

Chapter 1

A BRIEF HISTORY OF DIVORCE AND PARENT-CHILD CONTACT ISSUES

Child custody laws have changed throughout history. Societal opinions about marriage and childbearing, roles and responsibilities of parents, and adult beliefs about the best interests of children shift over time. Social norms affect our beliefs about children, parenting, and marriage, so it is not surprising that laws governing family life change over time. Currently, the Supreme Court's parental rights doctrine guides state child custody laws and decisions by making paramount the fundamental rights of parents to raise their children, and best interest doctrines issued by each state value the child's need to have contact with both parents after divorce. Parents are considered the best care givers for the child unless proven unfit, regardless of whether the child was born to parents who were married or not ("The Supreme Courts Parental Rights Doctrine," n.d.).

HISTORY OF CHILD CUSTODY

During the 16th century, English common law held that a child born out of wedlock was considered "*filius nullius,* a child of no family – allowing neither the mother nor father custodial rights" (Mason, 1994). Bastardly laws were established in England during the 1500's. They defined how children born out of wedlock were cared for and treated. Children were the community's responsibility and were often assigned as apprentices to poor families or shipped to the new American colonies as indentured servants.

Due to the growing number of illegitimate children being born and the increasing costs to raise them, a law was enacted that required the father of the child to contribute to the cost of raising the child (Teichman, 1982). Further laws were established to punish the mother of the child for having sexual relations outside of marriage (Zunshine, 2005). Children were viewed as property during this time, and their emotional needs for close and secure relationships with their parents were not necessarily considered when determining their care.

Some of these laws were carried over to the new American colonies developing in North America. The North American colonies needed workers to help build and expand the colonies; therefore, children being sent from England as indentured servants were of great benefit. They were not seen as children needing care and nurturance. They were seen as workers and treated harshly (Mason, 1994). Therefore, children's contact with parents was not a significant factor in decisions made by courts about a child's future.

English common law afforded women no legal rights to their children during marriage. Fathers held rights to the child and the child's earnings. As property, children belonged to the father and fathers could assign those rights (children) to an unrelated third-party if they so desired (Klaff, 1982). This was challenged in *de Manneville v. de Manneville* (1804) when the Court of the Chancery intervened in the father's legal right to custody of the child and returned the infant to its mother. The case was originally heard as *Rex v. de Manneville* by the Court of the King's Bench, which denied the mother's writ of habeas corpus to have the infant returned to her because they lacked the authority to change custody. The mother took her case to the Court of the Chancery where it was determined that it was best for the child to be with its mother. This was one of the first instances where the child's best interest to have consistent contact with a parent was the determining factor in a custody issue (Baker & Eichler, 2023).

Most of the new American colonies upheld English law and viewed children as property rights of the father. Divorce was rare during this time as English Canon law maintained that once married the marriage could not be destroyed. Colonies that followed English law rarely granted a divorce and when they did it usually did not allow for remarriage. Some colonies established more liberal laws and granted divorces for adultery, abandonment, and absence of economic support. However, divorces did not usually address children unless the child was the product of adultery, and the husband was asking for a divorce on those grounds. The absence of custodial issues during this time was most likely because women did not believe they could win custody and therefore never raised the issue, or they did not have to fight for custody because the father had deserted the family and left the children with the mother (Mason, 1994).

Reforms in English law allowing young children to remain with their mothers in instances of divorce occurred in the mid-nineteenth century and became known as the Tender Years' Doctrine. By 1873, the law reform included children up to 16 years of age and allowed the court of chancery to grant mothers custody or custodial time (Mason, 1994). The first case in America supporting the tender years doctrine was in 1813. A Pennsylvania court found that a mother should retain custody of her two daughters because she had been a good mother to the children, even though she violated Pennsylvania law and married her paramour while her ex-husband was still living (Commonwealth v. Addicks, 1813). In 1881, the Kansas Court stated that in custody issues, "above all things, the paramount consideration is, what will promote the welfare of the child" (Chapsky v. Wood, 1881).

Some scholars have stated that determining custodial issues based on the belief that children were best raised by their mothers originated in the 1800's as a reaction to child protection concerns. They believed that children's best interests were not being served by common law practices, which considered children as property and therefore belonging to the father (Klaff, 1982). As stated previously, children were being used as workers rather than being nurtured and protected during their early years. The importance of parental contact and custodial care became a focus in court decisions when parents were not married during the 19th century.

In 1973 a New York family court judge found that a presumptive preference for mothers violated fathers' fourteenth amendment of equal rights protections (People v. Watts, 1973), including the importance of the child's relationship with both parents in custodial decisions. Some states implemented a standard that custodial decisions requiring maternal custody absent a finding that the mother was unfit, was a violation of the equal rights amendment (Devine v. Devine, 1981). By 1981, 13 states were making custodial decisions based on best interest rather than the gender of the parent. Those critical of the best interest standard believed that it violated current child developmental knowledge that children benefitted most by mothers serving as the primary caretakers (Klaff, 1982).

Fathers arguing for equal rights and time with their children after divorce found themselves fighting deeply entrenched gender biases that mothers were somehow inherently better caregivers, particularly to young children. This spurred social science research in the 80's to test hypotheses about how children's wellbeing was affected by parenting time schedules after divorce (Warshak, 2017). After 30 years of research outcomes supporting the importance of father involvement after divorce and the positive effects that father involvement has on the long-term outcomes of children, legislative changes are now being made in some states that create a legal presumption of joint custody and equal physical custody between parents after divorce (National Parents Organization, 2019).

HISTORY OF PARENT-CHILD CONTACT ISSUES

Parents engaged in custody litigation during divorce are arguing for rights and time with their children. When society supports parental involvement during childhood and research has shown that children benefit from consistent contact with both parents after divorce, custody litigation may be likely if one parent opposes involvement of the other parent after divorce. High conflict divorce is characterized by prolonged litigation, high levels of hostility between the parents, and can leave emotional and psychological scars on parents and children. Children can get caught in the middle of warring parents, and their relationships with one or both parents can be negatively impacted (Bernet et al., 2016).

Mention of parent-child contact problems during separation and divorce began to appear in the writings of psychiatrists and psychologists in the 1940's. Lorandos (2020) provided a historical outline of these issues in his research article examining the extent of parental alienation in court cases from 1985-2018. The authors will follow and expand on that timeline here as it offers the most complete history they have found.

In 1943, child psychiatrist Daniel Levy described family dynamics in his book entitled *Maternal Overprotection,* where a child's negativity toward their father was caused by the mother's negativity about the father. In 1949, Wilhelm Reich discussed divorcing parents who were so consumed with a need to get revenge that they made false statements to the child about the other parent. This type of denigration created fear or anger in the child toward the parent and resulted in the child not wanting to spend time with the parent after the divorce. In 1953, psychiatrist Juliette Despert wrote about parents who retained the majority of possession time with children after divorce and negatively influenced the children's love for the other parent. She concluded that children were harmed by such behavior.

In the 1960's family therapists began dealing with parent-child contact problems in their therapy sessions. Murray Bowen (1961) developed theory and therapy techniques to work with the family system as opposed to individuals within the family. He described dynamics within families that interfered with healthy development. One dynamic he discussed was unhealthy alignments between parents and children. He described some parents as needing to create an overdependence between themselves and the child, causing a negative effect on the child's relationship with the other parent.

Another family therapist, Salvador Minuchin (1974), coined the term cross-generational coalition to describe alignments between one parent and the child that interfered in the child's relationship with the other parent. Minuchin discussed how this type of alignment "cuts off" the child's relationship with the other parent and leaves them in an almost equal position of power within the family as the parent. The child often feels empowered to make decisions about the amount of time they spend with their parents (Woodall & Woodall, 2017). Often, the child believes he/she is entitled to make such decisions because the favored parent has told the child that he/she should only have to see the other parent or go to the other parent's home by choice.

In these situations, the healthy family hierarchy which is commonly depicted as an inverted triangle (Diagram 1) with each parent at the top and the child at the bottom is instead depicted (Diagram 2) with the favored parent and the child at the top and the other parent at the bottom. The parent develops a coalition, in Minuchin's terms, with the child instead of the other parent.

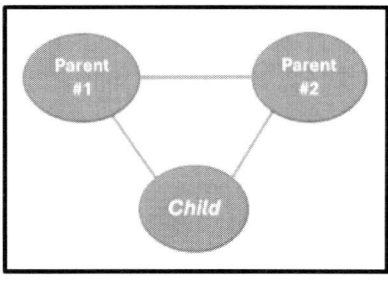
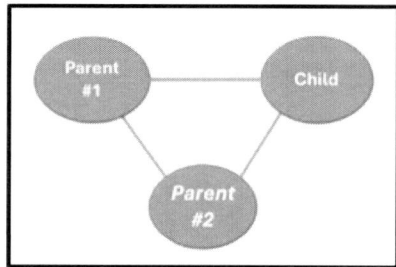

Diagram 1   Diagram 2

Judith Wallerstein and Joan Kelly (1976) conducted long-term research on 131 children from divorcing families. They documented results in some of the children where exclusive alignments were created between one of the parents and the child during the divorce process, which led to the child actively rejecting a relationship with the other parent. Some of the notable characteristics were that the rejection of the parent was fueled by the anger and hatred of the favored parent toward the other parent, and that the child had a previously positive relationship with the parent they were rejecting before the separation occurred.

Severe Contact Refusal

The 1980's produced several significant publications reflecting sociological and psychological findings that supported previous findings that children could be manipulated during divorce and separation to reject a once loved parent (Johnston et al., 1985; Benedek & Schetky, 1985; Gardner, 1985 & 1987). Johnston and her colleagues (1985), spoke to the tendency of these children to be severely polarized in their views of their parents. They idealized and adored one parent and despised and rejected the other parent. Benedek and Schetky (1985) described the child caught in a terrible loyalty bind, feeling pressured by one or both parents to dislike the other parent. They stated that the children could be influenced and eventually "brainwashed" to believe the negative commentary from one parent.

Parental Alienation

Richard Gardner, an adolescent psychiatrist working with high-conflict divorce, published his first writings (1985) on what came to be known as the Parental Alienation Syndrome (PAS). The characteristics of which echoed the other research findings occurring at this time. He noted that the children appeared to have a kind of mental obsession with hatred of one parent, while idealizing the other. Gardner discussed the brainwashing quality of the favored parent's messaging, reflected in the child's negative commentary and beliefs about the other parent.

In Gardner's 1992 book entitled *The Parental Alienation Syndrome*, he identified eight characteristics present in the child when PAS was likely the explanation for the child's resistance to one parent.

> (1) Campaign of denigration – represented by extreme hatred and vilification of the parent, although Gardner stated that he found the expressed hatred often combined with secretly held loving feelings of the parent. He wrote that the campaign of denigration was like a "litany," much of which was found to be unjustified or exaggerated. Gardner stated, "After minimal prompting by a lawyer, judge, or mental health professional, or other person involved in the litigation, the brain recording will be turned on, and a command performance is provided in which the targeted parent's defects are listed at length" (p. 77).
> (2) Weak, frivolous, and absurd rationalizations for the deprecation – represented by minor altercations between the child and the rejected parent, normal parenting failures that most children get over quickly, trivial request of the child by the rejected parent like brushing their teeth, or annoying behaviors of the parent that members of a family regularly deal with like snoring or eating too loudly.
> (3) Lack of ambivalence – represented by descriptions of the favored parent as all-good and descriptions of the targeted or rejected parent as all-bad.
> (4) The independent thinker phenomenon – represented by the child's adamant statements that they alone have decided to reject the parent, and that no other person has influenced their need to do so.
> (5) Reflexive support of the alienating parent – represented by the child supporting the alienating parent's views and opinions of the rejected parent, sometimes even more vociferously than the alienating parent. This characteristic can also be expressed in the child's refusal to accept evidence that their complaint about the rejected parent is inaccurate.
> (6) Absence of guilt over cruelty to and/or exploitation of the alienated parent – represented by a complete disregard for the rejected parent's feelings and an inability to acknowledge that what they are expecting

of the parent is unfair, often stating that they do not care if their words are hurtful to the parent. Gardner provided the example of a father being told by the child that he needed to continue financing their food, clothing, and private school education despite the fact that they did not want to see him until they were an adult.

(7) Presence of borrowed scenarios – represented by the child's litany of complaints sounding rehearsed and including adult language and/or stories of things that happened when the child was not present or was too young to have a memory about it.

(8) Spread of animosity to the extended family of the alienated parent – represented by the child rejecting grandparents, aunts, uncles, and cousins of the alienated parent. These relatives were people that the child previously spent time with and enjoyed positive relationships.

These characteristics have been shown to be unique characteristics of alienated children in 36 empirical studies (Harman et al., 2022). They are currently used in models of assessment for parental alienation (Baker, 2018; Bernet & Greenhill, 2021; Morrison & Ring, 2021). The authors will discuss the characteristics in several of the chapters in this book, and case examples will be offered to provide more detailed descriptions of how the characteristics may be present in a mental health professional's office.

Gardner suffered attacks from advocacy groups stating that he was discrediting abuse allegations made by children. Many critics have said that he self-published his work and, therefore, his work should not be viewed as credible. Gardner did self-publish some of his work, but he also published over twenty peer-reviewed journal articles in professional journals, and reviews of his books were published in peer-reviewed journals eleven times (warshak.com). The term PAS has been replaced with Parental Alienation (PA). It refers to one type of contact refusal that typically occurs within the context of a high-conflict separation or divorce when the child aligns with one parent and rejects the other (Bernet et al., 2016).

One of the largest studies to date documenting the capacity for children to be manipulated by a parent to fear, dislike, hate, and/or reject a parent was completed by Stanely Clawar and Brynne Rivlin, published initially by the American Bar Association in 1991 in a book entitled *Children Held Hostage.* The authors reviewed 700 cases of families involved in custody litigation and detailed the strategies used by parents that negatively influenced children's beliefs and perceptions about the other parent. The techniques used were described as programming and brainwashing techniques. In 2013, the authors published a second edition after reviewing 300 additional families, which further supported their original findings that children were being weaponized in custody battles and children could be convinced to reject a once-loved parent.

In 1993, Diedra Rand applied the term Munchausen Syndrome by Proxy (MSP) to describe alienating parents who used false abuse allegations during divorce litigation as a way to keep the child from the other parent and convince the child that the parent was dangerous. In the traditional use of the term, the parent, generally the mother, induces symptoms in their child or falsifies medical records to make the child appear to be suffering from some illness when examined by medical professionals. The mother is driven by the need to keep the child dependent on them and robs the child of normal developmental experiences. It is a severe form of emotional child abuse that can include physical abuse when the mother actually harms the child to create a symptom or wound and medical professionals attribute it to an illness.

Rand explained in her writings that originally, professionals thought MSP could only occur in younger children because as they aged, they would understand what the mother was doing to them and tell someone. However, researchers found many children aged and became duplicitous in falsifying symptoms to medical professionals. This was described as the mother and child developing a "folie a' deux" relationship about the child's false medical condition, where both parent and child expressed the belief that the child was truly ill. Rand applied the MSP diagnosis to parents (both mothers and fathers) who use sexual abuse allegations during separation and divorce to cease contact between the parent and the child. They interrogate the child after visits with the other parent, take the child to be examined or interviewed, and make allegations to child protective services and law enforcement that the parent has abused the child. Eventually, the child comes to believe the false narrative and refuses to see the other parent.

In the early 2000's children's resistance to a parent during separation and divorce was explained from a broader perspective, considering different levels of rejection and multiple factors influencing the child. Johnston and Kelly (2001) emphasized the need for mental health and legal professionals to recognize that all cases did not have the extreme components described by Gardner. They urged professionals to consider other causal factors outside of one parent's negative influence to explain the child's resistance to the parent. Johnston and Kelly referred to their findings as a "reformulation" of parental alienation (PA); however, their description of an alienated child as one who persistently expressed very strong negative opinions and beliefs about one parent that were disproportionate to the child's actual experience, seemed to echo the description provided by Gardner only using different words.

Pathological alienation was put forth by Richard Warshak (2003) to describe a child who shares one parent's negative view of the other parent and, as a result, exhibits extreme aversion to the parent with whom they once enjoyed a normal relationship. Nevertheless, PA came to be the term used by most legal and mental health professionals to refer to a situation where a child refuses contact with a parent due primarily to the alienating behaviors of the favored parent (Bernet et al., 2016).

Professionals working with divorcing families began writing more on the continuum of resistance in children and the continuum of parenting behaviors that could contribute to a child's reluctance to see the other parent, which led to an expansion of the terminology used and a deepened understanding of treatment options. While this was a necessary and ultimately helpful outgrowth of the scientific understanding of parent-child contact problems, it also served to confuse professionals and dilute the credibility of the term parental alienation. Nevertheless, the professionals working with these families needed to explore the varied contributing factors that could explain the many different levels of rejection observed in children.

In 2004, Leslie Drozd and Nancy Olesen published an article arguing for the importance of more complex, multivariate thinking in forensic evaluations. The authors put forth a model for decision-making to help forensic evaluators differentiate between estrangement (justified resistance to a parent), alienation, and abuse. They introduced the term counter-productive protective parenting, which was meant to describe a parent who engaged in behaviors that restricted the child's contact with the other parent during divorce because of their own heightened levels of anxiety, which were a reaction to their own experience of abuse with the other parent not to the child's experience of abuse.

In 2007, the concept of maternal gatekeeping during divorce was discussed in a journal article by Pruett and colleagues entitled, "The hand that rocks the cradle: Maternal gatekeeping after divorce." The authors describe maternal gatekeeping as behaviors and beliefs that interfere with collaborative parenting after divorce. In general, these behaviors limit the other parent's ability to be meaningfully and actively involved in the child's life. Mothers may be motivated by their own belief that the other parent is not competent, which may or may not be accurate, their need to maintain control, their own personal insecurities, anger at the other parent, and or their need to maintain pre-divorce parenting roles and dynamics.

In 2010, Steven Friedlander and Majorie Walters published an article describing their treatment with children who were exhibiting "resistance and refusal" behaviors toward a parent during divorce. Their work has provided broader treatment goals based on an assessment of the multiple factors causing the child's resistance and advocates for the use of multiple providers working as a team (Walters & Friedlander, 2016; Johnston et al., 2001). The term "resist-refusal" dynamics was a result of their work over the last 25 years. Their treatment team model is discussed in Chapter 11 of this book.

In 2013, there was consideration by APA for inclusion of parental alienation in the DSM-5 as a mental disorder. The ultimate decision was not to include the term but instead include a diagnosis called "Child Affected by Parental Relationship Distress (CAPRD)" (APA, 2013). The diagnostic term is used to describe a continuum of reactions that a child may have because of parental discord, including realistic estrangement, loyalty binds, and parental alienation (Bernet et al., 2016). Two of the authors of the DSM explained in an article written with Dr. William Bernet (2016), that the decision not to include parental alienation was based on the work group's belief that:

> Parental alienation is a term more frequently used in forensic settings ... to determine a more objective truth than what practicing clinicians are asked to assess. Practicing clinicians deal with the beliefs of the child and know that there may be distortions in those beliefs, but seldom are allowed the intense evaluation of forensic mental health experts... For this reason, the Relational Processes Work group recommended ... to use the appropriate broader category, that is, CAPRD, parent-child relational problem (PCRP), and/or child psychological abuse. (pp. 575-576)

In 2017, the American Professional Society on the Abuse of Children (APSAC) found that children severely affected by parental alienation had experienced child maltreatment. Alienating behaviors that altered the child's perceptions and memories of a parent were found to meet the criteria of child psychological abuse (APSAC, 2017). In 2018, Harman and colleagues identified alienating behaviors as a form of family violence when children are weaponized to control the other parent, limit the parent's freedom, and/or threaten and intimidate the parent.

After years of social science research, professional consensus about terminology and assessment is surfacing. In 2021, Bernet and colleagues conducted a survey of custody evaluators regarding terminology for parent-child contact issues during divorce and separation. They found almost 90% of custody evaluators agreed that the term "contact refusal referred to a child's resistance or rejection to contact or relationship with a parent" and that the term represented a broad concept that could be caused by many different variables. Eighty percent of the respondents agreed that parental alienation was "one type of contact refusal." And that PA was a situation where the child was aligned with one parent and rejected the other. There was 80% agreement on the eight characteristics originally defined by Gardner; 90% agreement on the definition of alienating behaviors as referring to the behaviors of the alienating parent that cause the child's rejection of the parent; 90% agreement that the definition of "alienating parent" referred to the parent engaging in alienating behaviors; 80% agreement that the term alienated parent referred to the parent whom the child was rejecting; and 85% agreement on the definitions and differentiation between mild, moderate, and severe levels of alienation. These terms will be discussed in further detail throughout this book.

Parent-child contact problems have been described, explored, and researched over the last 50-plus years. Our ability to identify them accurately, assess their level of significance, evaluate the multiple causes, develop treatment plans, and implement those plans has evolved over time. The literature on parental alienation has reached a mature stage (Harman et al., 2023), where there are more quantitative studies and research driven by theory. Therefore, the value of this book is in coalescing all that has come before us to understand how children come to resist parents during divorce and how we, as clinicians, can help families struggling to maintain close attachments and relationships through times of transition and change.

Chapter 2

CAUSES OF PARENT-CHILD CONTACT ISSUES

> **Learning Objectives:**
> 1. Understand how loyalty conflicts originate and can cause contact issues.
> 2. Understand the impact of pre- and post-divorce conflict and interpersonal conflict on contact issues.
> 3. Understand the impact of different characteristics of the parent and child on contact issues.
> 4. Understand the impact of family dynamics on contact issues.

One of the first things to consider when working with a family experiencing parent-child contact problems is how the family arrived at this state of dysfunction in the first place. You may feel overwhelmed as each person comes into your office with their side of the story thinking you may never get to the bottom of what is actually happening. Unfortunately, this investigation does not usually provide quick answers. You will need to consider multiple hypotheses when working with these families and be careful not to get "sucked in" to one idea too quickly. Be open to alternative explanations as you work with the family. To help in your understanding of the dynamics, it is essential to include a thorough screening and evaluation of the behaviors of each parent and each of the children. This process should also consider the many interconnected familial and individual factors of family conflict and abuse. Additionally, you will need to differentiate between various types and the different levels of severity of parent-child contact problems that you may encounter (Drozd et al., 2013; Johnston et al., 2005; Saunders & Faller, 2016).

In the more severe cases where a child is outright rejecting all contact with a parent, a key foundation of treatment is determining the child's route to resistance (Woodall & Woodall, 2017; Fidler et al., 2013). Once a therapist understands the pathway the child took to decide that rejecting a parent was the best way to survive, a therapist can guide them to a different pathway where the child is not sacrificing a relationship with a "good enough" parent.

Likewise, the same information is useful to a clinician working with a child who has not come to the point of completely rejecting a parent yet is still showing some distress with the conflict between the parents. In some cases, a child may progress from mildly rejecting a parent to refusing all contact with that parent. If you are working with the family and witness the child's change in stance towards that parent, you may have a better understanding of what factors contributed to it. Understanding these many factors contributing to a child's resistance or refusal to see a parent, significantly aid the clinician in navigating and addressing parent-child contact issues.

Many researchers have spent considerable time and effort studying why a child might resist or refuse one of their parents following a divorce (Kelly & Johnston, 2001; Johnston, 2005; Bernet, 2006; Friedlander & Walters, 2010; Fidler & Bala, 2020; Johnston & Sullivan, 2020). These reasons can be categorized broadly into circumstances surrounding the divorce, parental conflict pre- and post-separation, parent factors, child factors, and overall family dynamics. In the sections to come, we'll delve into some of the theories and research findings to consider as you work with these families and try to determine what factors are at play.

Loyalty Conflicts

It is typical for a child from a divorced home to miss their mom while at their dad's house and vice versa. Having some degree of discomfort can be normal. Loyalty conflicts occur when a child tries to maintain positive feelings toward both parents even though the parents are hostile toward each other (Bernet et al., 2016). However, one or both parents can intensify this loyalty conflict by pressuring a child to support that parent's side in disagreements with the other parent. Parents may also seek emotional support from the child, confiding in them or seeking validation for their feelings or decisions. Maybe a parent tells the child something like, "You understand why I had to leave, right?" The child now feels like they must validate that parent's perspective. When the child feels that their loyalty to one parent conflicts with their loyalty to the other, they are constantly in emotional distress (Freeman, 2020). In divorce, understanding the complex nature of loyalty binds is essential. The adversarial process inherent in a divorce may promote the idea that a child must pick which parent is "right," especially if the parents involve them in their conflict. Such loyalty bonds can profoundly impact the child, negatively affecting their emotional health and relationships with both parents.

A child experiencing distress due to a loyalty conflict may attempt to resolve it by resisting contact with a parent. Cognitive dissonance is a psychological tension resulting from holding two conflicting ideas simultaneously (Festinger, 1957). Individuals experiencing cognitive dissonance are highly motivated to reduce the stress it causes.

For example, a child dealing with the cognitive dissonance of trying to love two parents who hate each other may resolve this tension by rejecting one of their parents (Freeman, 2020). They may feel guilty when spending time with one parent and not the other, leading them to potentially avoid contact with one parent so they do not hurt the other parent's feelings. Once they have ceased contact with a parent, they will often report to you that they feel much better and have less stress and anxiety.

Upon hearing this, some therapists may believe that this is a good solution for the child; however, this solution leads to long-term psychological issues in the child. Such an outright refusal of contact demonstrates that the initial loyalty conflict has evolved into a situation where the child is now alienated from the parent (Bernet et al., 2016). If you can identify how each parent is creating a loyalty bind with the child, it can direct your treatment with the parents as you educate them on how their behaviors are causing stress to their child.

Reactions to Circumstances of Divorce

Sometimes, a child's refusal to interact with one parent after a divorce can be a response to specific situations related to the separation. For example, a child could feel angry or hurt by how one parent decided to end the marriage and leave the family. The way the parent handled the separation could have caused emotional pain, leading the child to withdraw from them. Even if the parents planned the separation, the child's experience may appear abrupt and as if one parent just left.

A child might also disapprove of a parent's actions or behavior, whether related to the divorce or other aspects of life. This disapproval can make it hard for them to want to spend time with this parent. Similarly, if the child feels sympathy or pity for the other parent—perhaps they believe this parent was wronged in the divorce—they might show favoritism towards this parent (Johnston, 2005).

Parental Conflict Pre- and Post Separation

Loyalty conflicts are more likely if the child has been exposed to conflict pre- and post-divorce. Different factors regarding the conflictual relationship between the parents can contribute to a child's resistance or refusal to see a parent. If children were aware of the conflict between their parents before the separation, what they observed and experienced would impact how they viewed each parent (Fidler & Bala, 2020).

If the conflict continues in the co-parenting relationship or if the communication between the parents is poor, it could also impact the child's willingness to engage with both parents. Suppose the parents continue to have conflict with one another. In that case, the child will likely be exposed to it, and the child will have to put increasing emotional energy into maintaining a relationship with both parents. The emotional stress this puts on the child can lead to rejection of one parent, as described in the loyalty conflicts section.

Intimate Partner Violence/Domestic Violence

A child can be significantly harmed if exposed to substantial or persistent conflict between the parents (El Sheikh et al., 2008; McTavish et al., 2016). Intimate partner violence is the physical, sexual, or psychological harm caused by a current or former partner (Centers for Disease Control and Prevention, 2009). Domestic violence is physical, sexual, or emotional maltreatment by one family member to another, and it includes all types of family violence (American Psychological Association, 1996). Most professionals agree that it is imperative to screen for abuse and IPV in family courts (Hamel & Baker, 2022).

Sometimes the child has witnessed some of the intimate partner violence, and that affects who they blame for the loss of the family.

When a child is expected to spend time with a parent they witnessed abusing their other parent, they may experience a range of conflicting emotions. The child will be torn between their natural attachment to both parents along with the fear, confusion, or even guilt associated with the abusive parent's actions. The child may also feel torn between loyalty to both parents. They may feel pressure to show allegiance to the abusive parent to avoid upsetting them, while, at the same time, feel the need to protect or support the victimized parent.

When there has been substantial documentation of IPV, it is understandable that the victim parent will be cautious in coparenting with the perpetrator. Safeguards may need to be put in place for the victims. The Court may not expect victims of IPV to be friendly coparents, and the Court must consider these factors when putting orders in place that dictate joint interactions with the parents. Past IPV will be relevant to future co-parenting (Austin & Drozd, 2013). IPV may also be on a continuum and can impact how well the parents can work together. There is a difference between a single episode or intermittent episodes of mild violence (e.g., pushing, slamming doors, throwing a phone, etc.) between partners and chronic, calculated, and escalated episodes of violence between the partners (Heyman et al., 2013), with the latter being more harmful and less treatable.

While in some cases, IPV is not properly identified, there are also cases where children are influenced to falsely believe that a parent is dangerous or a parent has inappropriately shared details of the intimate partner violence (Fidler & Bala, 2020; Harman & Matthewson, 2020). The child may be led to believe that the other parent has committed acts of physical, emotional, or sexual abuse when no such abuse has occurred, or the severity of actions may be exaggerated. Even if the child has never experienced direct harm, being told that the other parent has abused them or could harm them in the future may instill fear. The child may start to see the accused parent as dangerous or threatening and mistrust the accused parent.

Case Vignette: Mary

Mary was 13 when her parents separated. She had an older brother, Eddie, who was 18, and a younger sister, Stephanie, who was 8. Eddie and Mary were aware of the tension between their parents, and they had seen their parents yell at each other and push each other around at times, with both parents being aggressive. One day, Mary's mom picked Eddie, Mary, and Stephanie up from school with all their belongings in the car and told them they were moving to their uncle's house to get away from their dad. Mary's mom had a serious conversation with the kids to let them know that she had to leave because their father had threatened her with her life and had beaten her many times over the years. She gave them many details of their physical fights, including sharing with the children that their dad had raped her. When they were at their uncle's house, she told them not to let their father know where they were as she feared for her safety.

The kids did not see their father for months until their mom filed for divorce, and the court set a visitation plan. At that time, Mary refused to see her father. Stephanie was hesitant, but she would go. Eddie was allowed to do what he wanted due to his age, but he did maintain a relationship with his father. He did not quite believe everything his mom had told them, as he perceived his father as the more passive of the two parents.

This is a case where if there was IPV, the mom inappropriately shared details with the children, which undermined their relationship with their father. Fortunately, Eddie was not as influenced, but Mary no longer wanted to be with her father, whom she perceived now as a dangerous man.

Parent Characteristics

Characteristics of each parent, such as mental health, negative behaviors, personality, and parenting style, may also facilitate resistance/refusal (Fidler & Bala, 2020). Many researchers have focused on the characteristics of the favored parent's psychopathology and personality disorders. Favored parents tend to present themselves favorably, have rigid moral values, and are more sensitive to criticism. These parents often use primitive defenses to justify and perpetuate the alienation of the other parent (Gordon et al., 2008; Roma et al., 2021; Verrocchio et al., 2018). These defense mechanisms help them manage their feelings of inadequacy, jealousy, or anger, and they project these emotions onto the targeted parent. Here are some common primitive defenses used by favored parents:

- Projection—Attributing their own unacceptable feelings and thoughts to the other parent. An alienating parent may accuse the other parent of being neglectful or abusive, projecting their own hostile or controlling behaviors onto the other parent.
- Splitting—Viewing people and situations in black-and-white terms, as all good or all bad. The alienating parent may idealize themselves

as the perfect parent and demonize the target parent as entirely bad and worthless as a parent. When alienating parents teach children to see others in black-and-white terms as entirely good or entirely bad, and rationalize unfair treatment of others, it undermines the children's ability to form healthy intimate relationships.

- Denial—Refusing to acknowledge undesired realities. A favored parent may deny the child's need for a relationship with the other parent, insisting that the child is better off without them despite evidence to the contrary.
- Projective Identification—Projecting unwanted feelings onto another person and interacting in a way that makes the person conform to these projections. A preferred parent may treat the other parent as hostile or dangerous, which can provoke frustration or defensive behaviors from the targeted parent, seemingly validating the alienator's projections.
- Dissociation—Detaching from reality to avoid experiencing distressing thoughts or feelings. An alienating parent might dissociate from their own feelings of guilt or responsibility in the breakdown of the relationship, blaming the other parent entirely.
- Acting Out—Expressing unconscious emotional conflicts through actions rather than words. The alienating parent may engage in manipulative behaviors, such as making false allegations or interfering with visitation schedules, to act out their underlying anger and resentment.
- Rationalization—Justifying irrational or unacceptable behavior with logical reasons. The favored parent may rationalize their behavior by claiming they are acting in the child's best interest, even when their actions are clearly harmful to the child's relationship with the other parent.

Both favored parents and rejected parents can exhibit some rigidity. A parent's rigidity can impede the parent's ability to maintain empathy and focus on the child's needs and well-being. The inflexible parent is unable to consider alternative viewpoints and will often become entrenched in their distorted perceptions, which often leads to emotional dysregulation. Difficulty in managing emotions can result in exaggerated responses and unnecessary drama, affecting both the children and the other parent (Walters & Friedlander, 2016).

Roma et al. (2021) found that the profiles of rejected fathers suggest that they may demonstrate a lack of energy to deal with issues as well as an overall depressive mood state. Many of them tended to be more introverted and had adapted to the high levels of conflict they experienced with their child's mother.

In some hybrid cases, the rejected parent often plays a significant role in the resist-refuse dynamic. The rejected parent is already distressed by the rejection of their child. At the same time, the rejected parent may believe their parenting is superior to the favored parent's parenting. Sometimes, this parent will overcompensate for the perceived deficiencies of the favored parent, perhaps by adding more restrictions to what the child is allowed to do, which can lead to even more extreme behaviors than usual, further aggravating their issues with the child. When the case involves a teenager, this overcompensating can even cause more issues in the parent-child relationship as the teen is requiring increasing independence (Walters & Friedlander, 2016).

Attachment

Attachment is an emotional connection that develops between a child and a caregiver based on the caregiver's ability to respond sensitively to the child's need for security (Bowlby, 1969). This bond is fundamental in shaping the child's social, emotional, and cognitive development. When a child is younger, the child seeks the proximity of an attachment figure in times of fear or perceived danger (Main et al., 2011).

Following a divorce, the attachment between a child and parent is an especially critical aspect of the child's emotional and psychological well-being. The disruptions that accompany a divorce can significantly challenge the stability of the parent-child bond. Despite the change in family dynamics, maintaining a secure attachment with both parents is essential for the child's sense of security and later individuation and independence (Main et al., 2011).

The way parents handle the divorce and their ongoing relationship with their children plays an important role in mitigating the potential negative impact on the child. Consistent and loving communication, reassurance, and spending quality time with the child can help reinforce their sense of being valued and loved. Unfortunately, sometimes a child's attachment to both parents is corrupted by negative parental behaviors following a divorce (Baker & Eichler, 2016).

Child Characteristics

When evaluating parent-child contact issues, it is essential to consider the child's characteristics. These include the child's age and developmental stage, which can greatly influence their understanding and reaction to the contact situation. Cognitive abilities are also significant, as you determine how well the child can process and comprehend their circumstances.

The child's vulnerability and resilience must be assessed to understand how they may cope with the emotional challenges of contact (or not having contact with a parent). Additionally, the child's overall temperament affects how they interact with each parent. Finally, any special needs the child may have should be carefully considered in seeing how they play into the parent-child contact challenges (Fidler & Bala, 2020). For example, a child on the autism spectrum may be more impacted by parenting time schedules and inconsistencies between the homes than a neurotypical child.

Age/Developmental Preferences

Normal developmental preferences can play a big role in a child's behavior following a divorce. For instance, a child may feel more comfortable and secure around the parent who has been their primary caregiver as they've likely spent more time with this parent and have built a strong bond with them.

If the child is on the younger side, they might experience separation anxiety during transitions between parents. This is a common part of childhood development where a child can feel distressed when they're not with their primary caregiver. This could make them more resistant to spending time with the other parent.

Another developmental factor could be that the child identifies more with one parent due to shared interests or gender (Johnston, 2005; Friedlander & Walters, 2010). For example, a daughter might feel more connected to her mother because they both enjoy thrift shopping or a son might feel a stronger bond with his father because of his love for football. This is not a divorce-specific phenomenon, as it also occurs in intact families (Friedlander & Walters, 2010).

As kids get older, practical reasons can also influence their decision. They might refrain from spending time with one parent to avoid disruptions to their school schedule or social activities. Or they might find one parent's household boring compared to the other (Johnston, 2005). All these factors can contribute to a child's resistance to spending time with one parent after a divorce.

Lastly, it's also possible that a child might prefer to spend time with the parent who places fewer demands on them and offers more benefits (Johnston, 2005). This could mean that the parent doesn't enforce as many rules, or maybe they allow more screen time or give the child more treats. However, it's important to remember that what might seem like a 'better deal' for the child in the short term might not necessarily be what's best for their development and well-being in the long run.

Case Vignette: Mackenzie

> Mackenzie's parents had been divorced since she was three. Her dad moved to a nearby town 45 minutes away. While she grew up in the tension of both parents really disliking each other, she had little difficulty going back and forth between households until middle school. In middle school, she started to want to get involved in more activities. Looking back, she would admit that part of the reason she wanted to be so involved in school was to escape the constant "drama" she would have to deal with when hearing about the frequent conflict between her two parents from her mom. Ironically, as she chose to escape more in school, it became more difficult for her to go to her dad's house. He would resent all of the things that were scheduled on "his time." His complaining about her schedule started leading to Mackenzie's resistance to going to his house until she refused to go altogether. After missing a summer with her dad, family therapy was ordered for her and her dad.

It was the job of the family therapist to disentangle all the players' roles in this dynamic, as they all contributed to Mackenzie's resistance to going to her dad's house. At first glance, knowing that Mackenzie was refusing to go to her dad's house, it may have appeared that Mackenzie was unjustly rejecting her dad. However, once the clinician started working with each person individually (including their mom) and obtained a history of the case, it became apparent that Mackenzie was not irrationally rejecting her dad but just wanting to be a teen and avoid the constant conflict between her parents.

Vulnerability/Resilience

Child resilience refers to a child's ability to recover from or adjust to change. It's the capacity to bounce back from stressful challenges and adapt to adversity. Resilience is a combination of personal characteristics, learned behaviors, and social support systems that enable a child to face challenges effectively. When parents divorce, children must adapt to many changes in their lives, and how well they manage the new situation has quite a bit to do with how resilient and how vulnerable they are.

Researchers have identified specific emotional vulnerabilities in children who reject a parent. These vulnerabilities often involve avoidance-based coping mechanisms and a reduced capacity for realistic relationships with others. While these vulnerabilities may not be obvious at first, the long-term effects of internalizing their distress and not addressing their unresolved grief over the loss of their intact family can manifest later in their relationships and self-esteem (Johnston et al., 2005). As their rejection of a parent continues, their social skills and emotional maturity will also continue to lag behind that of their peers and negatively impact their ability to have strong peer relationships.

Stubborn Child

Certain children have a natural tendency to resist change, a trait that can be particularly pronounced when their home environment undergoes significant shifts. They may have had a good attachment to both parents prior to the separation but then became very upset upon the divorce (Bernet, 2006). Usually, parents are aware of a child's resistance to change, but they still may be surprised by a child starting to resist or refuse contact with a parent due to the child's inflexibility. A child may also simply have some emotional distress that is beyond their abilities to cope. The child may also have oppositional traits that have manifested in other situations that make them generally resistant to any type of change. This can be a key factor to consider, especially if it is noted that the parents are behaving appropriately and doing their best to manage the situation in a thoughtful manner (Freeman, 2020).

Anxiety or Depression

Certain children may have a predisposition towards anxiety and depression, making them more susceptible to emotional distress. For these children, navigating the considerable stress and changes accompanying parental separation can be particularly challenging (Bernet, 2006). Their ability to cope with such a massive life change can vary widely and depends heavily on several factors.

One of the most significant factors is the nature of the relationship between the parents after the separation. If the parents maintain a cooperative and respectful relationship, the child will likely find it easier to adjust to the new family structure. On the other hand, if the parents' relationship is fraught with conflict, hostility, or a lack of communication, the child's stress levels may be exacerbated, and their ability to adapt could be severely hindered (Freeman, 2020).

FAMILY DYNAMICS

Unhealthy Alignments

Alignments within the extended family and with community professionals can also contribute to a child's resist/refuse behaviors toward a parent (Fidler & Bala, 2020). These alliances often create an environment where the child feels validated and is even encouraged to reject one parent. Ryan Thomas, a formerly alienated child, refers to the family members who sided with his preferred parent as "the regime" (Ryan Thomas Speaks, 205). This term underscores the powerful influence such collective support can have on a child's perceptions and attitudes toward a parent.

Triangulation

Triangulation in a family occurs when a third party is drawn into the relationship of two people in conflict. This third person can be another family member, a friend, or even a therapist. While triangulation can provide short-term relief from conflict, as the focus shifts from the original problem to the third party, it does not resolve the underlying issues and can create additional problems.

A common example in the context of divorce is when parents are in conflict, and one or both parents involve a child to take sides or perhaps even serve as a mediator. This parent behavior ruptures a proper parent-child relationship boundary as it creates an alliance between the child and a parent at the expense of the child's relationship with the other parent. This triangulates the relationship as the child is now in the middle of the parents' conflicted relationship rather than being outside and separate from it (Baker & Eichler, 2016). The triangulation creates much emotional distress for the child, who is now in an untenable position.

Sometimes, the child will attempt to triangulate a parent by complaining about the other parent. If they can get their mom to engage with them when they complain about their dad, or vice versa, they can feel they are a team. This can give the child a sense of power and can create some issues in all the relationships.

Enmeshment

While separation anxiety is normal in young children, it can be an indicator of pathological attachment to the favored parent when the child is older (Garber, 2004; Johnston et al., 2005). In these cases, only the favored parent can calm the child's anxieties. On the other hand, the child may be meeting the needs of the favored parent who is anxious or depressed without the child. Sometimes it is really difficult to say which came first—the child's anxieties or the parents. In your office, however, the resistance to leaving the favored parent may be blamed on the target parent's behaviors rather than the anxiety the child feels when leaving the favored parent.

This dynamic can evolve into an enmeshment between the child and the favored parent. In such a relationship, the psychological boundaries between the child and the parent are blurred or haven't been properly established. At first glance, this might appear to be a close and even desirable relationship, characterized by shared experiences and a strong bond (Friedlander & Walters, 2010).

One sign of such an enmeshed relationship that you may notice is the use of the collective pronoun "we" by either the favored parent or the child when describing personal experiences, feelings, or opinions. This suggests a lack of distinction between the individual experiences of the parent and child. The child's physical closeness to the preferred parent during therapy sessions, such as sitting unusually close or even on the parent's lap, could also indicate an enmeshed relationship (Friedlander & Walters, 2010).

Typically, a child in an enmeshed relationship is highly sensitive to the parent's emotional needs and may feel obligated to protect or take care of the parent. Often, neither the child nor the parent is aware of the unhealthy dynamics at play, believing instead that they simply share a close bond. In extreme cases, there might even be a clear role reversal where the child, rather than the parent, becomes the primary caregiver in the relationship, or parentification.

Parentification can be in a more practical form where the child assumes a parent's daily tasks and responsibilities such as cooking, cleaning, and taking care of younger siblings. The other form of parentification is more emotional, where the child is providing emotional support to the parent, acting as a confidant or therapist. Regardless of what form the parentification takes, this role corruption can be harmful to the child's development and well-being, negatively impacting his peer relationships and ability to make and maintain a healthy relationship with the other parent as they feel an obligation to stay with the preferred parent (Garber, 2011; Friedlander & Walters, 2010).

Another dynamic that impedes the child's development is infantilization, where the child is discouraged from achieving developmentally appropriate milestones of independence. The infantilizing parent needs to be needed, and when the child is young, that parent is viewed as a loving caretaker. However, as the child gets older, the parent will appear to be overprotective, overinvolved, and intrusive. The child will be discouraged from making friends and participating in extracurricular activities (Garber, 2011). You may hear different stories from each parent—the infantilizing parent may describe the child as regressed and needy, while the other parent will describe the child as behaving in a more age-appropriate manner at their house (Garber, 2011; Friedlander & Walters, 2010). In all forms of enmeshment, the parent-child relationship is mainly serving the favored parent's needs, and it significantly impedes the child's healthy development (Walters & Friedlander, 2016).

Parental Alienation

Parental alienation is a term used when a parent (alienating or favored parent) has undermined the child's relationship with the other parent (rejected or target parent) (Bernet, 2006). In pure cases of parental alienation, the primary reason for the child's rejection of the target parent is due to the influence of the favored parent. While some claim that parental alienation is just a belief system rather than science (Mercer, 2021), overwhelming research negates this claim (Harman et al., 2022). Saini et al. (2016) found agreement in the research about the alienating strategies that damage the relationship between the child and the target parent as well as typical behaviors that an alienated child exhibits.

When assessing a case for possible parental alienation, you must look for any potential alienating behaviors displayed by the parent(s). Alienating behaviors interfere in the child's relationship with the other parent and can alter the child's feelings and perceptions of the parent. They include but are not limited to bad-mouthing, denigration, limiting contact with the child, and inciting anger and fear in the child toward the parent. Chapter 4 provides a complete list of 17 alienating behaviors and describes them in detail. While a clinician may not always have access to all the pertinent information, any available evidence can prove valuable in differentiating the case. It is best not to rely solely on parent interviews for information. Assessment is discussed in more detail in the next chapter.

Sometimes if alienating behaviors are present, the evidence can be found in multiple places. Parents who claim that certain behaviors are occurring will often be able to provide supporting documentation. Text message exchanges between family members, emails sent within the family, notes or letters written by the children, and correspondence with teachers or other professionals can all provide valuable insights into the family dynamics. Reports from child protection services or medical and therapy records can also provide helpful information (Harman & Matthewson, 2020).

Alienating behaviors vary from mild forms of bad-mouthing to more severe controlling behaviors that ultimately can result in a child's complete refusal of contact with the target parent. Some parents may be alienating occasionally, maybe just when in heightened periods of stress, while others may constantly denigrate the other parent. The alienating behaviors can range from verbal cues, such as a tone of voice that indicates disgust when talking about the target parent, to more subtle nonverbal signs, like rolling their eyes or disengaging from the interaction when the other parent is mentioned. There are no gender differences in who is more likely to be the favored parent or target parent. However, the parent who has primary custody is usually the perpetrator of the alienating behaviors (Baker & Eichler, 2016; Harman et al., 2018).

Other complex dynamics can also increase the chances of a child rejecting a parent. For example, the parent may portray themselves as an underdog to the child in the conflict between the favored parent and target parent, and the child may feel the need to protect the favored parent. To maintain the protective stance, they may avoid expressing any positive feelings they may have towards the target parent. The child may also fear rejection or anger from the favored parent if they express positive feelings for the target parent, so it is safer for them to not to have positive feelings (Friedlander & Walters, 2010).

When a child is alienated, they feel completely justified in rejecting that parent. Their rejection often comes with a sense of self-righteousness. If you challenge their reasons for rejecting the parent, the child will often escalate their negative statements about that parent and react with even more intensity. Alienated children are very resistant to the belief that their rationale for rejecting that parent may be exaggerated (Woodall & Woodall, 2017).

Estrangement

At times, a parent may engage in harmful behaviors that cause a child to become estranged from them. Behaviors include being neglectful or abusive. The child may become estranged from a parent due to that parent's actions, which may have caused the child to withdraw from them entirely. Parents suffering from substance abuse or mental health issues that prohibit them from being able to adequately care for their child create rational concerns about their parenting capacity (Woodall & Woodall, 2017). As stated previously, the child may have witnessed family violence. If the parent left the family, the child could be struggling with feelings of abandonment and feel anxiety about being alone with the parent (Johnston, 2005). In these cases, the child's resistance is primarily due to the rejected parent's actions. The favored parent in these situations may be concerned about the child having contact with the other parent for a real reason, and the subsequent gatekeeping of that parent may seem, at first glance, to be undermining the child's relationship with the rejected parent.

These issues are often disputed and can cause significant distress and conflict within the family. However, the child's behaviors can provide important clues for you to determine if the child is more estranged than alienated. Usually, if a child is withdrawing due to harmful actions from a parent, the child will initially blame themselves before deciding that the parent is to blame. This self-blaming phase may delay the child's outright rejection of the parent. Also, if there is truth to the parent's behaviors damaging the relationship, you will likely have other people who have observed these behaviors and not just the favored parent (Woodall & Woodall, 2017).

Parental Alienation/Estrangement–Hybrid Case

There are some instances where a parent's behaviors may be problematic, but then a favored parent magnifies the negative impact of those behaviors, increasing the child's frustration with that parent. In those cases, the child may present as if they are more alienated than estranged. Such cases are a hybrid case of alienation—the target parent has contributed to some of the child's negative feelings towards them (Friedlander & Walters, 2010). For instance, maybe a parent had a substance abuse problem for a few years after a major stressor. During those years, the parent would be emotionally abusive to the child when intoxicated. Then, the parent realized the harm and sought treatment and stopped drinking altogether. However, the other parent continues to make a big deal of the incidents, perhaps even suggesting that the parent can never really change. The parent did engage in harmful parenting behaviors, but the child's rejection is out of proportion because there have not been substance abuse issues for a long time. Most children can deal with parent failures, especially when the parent has acknowledged them and altered behaviors.

Many post-divorce family dynamics might seem, at first glance, to be solely a matter of parental alienation. However, upon closer examination, these situations often reveal themselves to be much more complex. This underscores the importance of a comprehensive assessment into the causes of the contact problems. The vignettes below illustrate how a similar negative parental behavior can produce two different reactions in children.

Case Vignette: Emily and Jacob

Emily (15) and Jacob (12) primarily live with their mom, Laura. One weekend when they were with their mom, their dad was arrested for possession of cocaine. When Laura found out about their dad's arrest, she felt like she had to tell the children that their dad had chosen cocaine over them. She then prevented them from seeing their dad in the subsequent week and continued talking with them about how bad his choices were, leading the children to believe that their dad was not coming to see them and continuing to choose cocaine use over them.

Once their dad, Mark, went through the court process to see the children again, they were very angry at him for what they perceived as him abandoning them. Their mom continued to make negative remarks about their dad, saying that he would never change and that he would always be choosing his addiction over his children.

In the above case, while their dad's cocaine use would have caused some relationship issues between Emily and Jacob and their dad once they knew about it, the issues were made much bigger by how their mom framed the infraction as well as how she continued to talk about it when they did not have contact with their dad.

Case Vignette: Hailey and Hannah

Hailey and Hannah are 13-year-old twin sisters living with their mother, Sarah, following their parents' amicable divorce two years ago. Their father, David, has joint custody, and the girls spend every other weekend at his place. His parents live nearby, so sometimes they go to their grandparents' house on their weekends with him.

One weekend, while staying at their dad's, Hailey and Hannah noticed their father behaving unusually. They knew that their dad had a history of drug use as his intermittent use is what they blamed for their parents' divorce. While in his bathroom, they discovered a small bag containing a white powder hidden behind some toiletries. Realizing it was cocaine, they became alarmed. They called their mom, and she picked them up immediately. Their dad let them go without an argument.

Their mom later talked with the girls about how addiction can take hold of a person, and let them know that their dad loved them, but he sometimes struggled with his desire to alter how he felt. The girls were upset with their dad for doing that when they were there. They were worried about going back, but they later told their mom they would feel all right going back as long as they were staying at their grandparents' house with their dad so if he did it again, they would not be alone.

In this case, the mom did more to protect the children's relationship with their dad so they did not become as angry with him. Although they did have some fear about going to see him again, their fear was realistic, and they were able to think of a solution to help them feel safe while maintaining their attachment to their dad.

Family of Origin Issues

Sometimes, one of the driving factors for the contact issues is more unconscious and hidden. A parent may be reenacting their own childhood trauma of parental loss or feelings of abandonment; that is, there is an unconscious repetition of traumatic experiences from one's past in present-day relationships. This psychological phenomenon is a way for individuals to process unresolved trauma, but as it plays out, it can inadvertently perpetuate harmful patterns within the family.

The clinician at the intake can look for signs of this when asking screening questions about each of the parent's family of origin. It is not unusual in this process to find a disruption in the relationship between a favored parent and one of their parents that happened at the child's current age that the favored parent's child is now experiencing contact issues with a target parent. Or, conversely, for the reenactment of a trauma to be created on the target parent's side.

To work with unprocessed trauma, the clinician will need to help the favored parent see the repetition of the past into the present (Fraiberg et al., 1975). Woodall and Woodall (2017) refer to this as transgenerational haunting, a psychoanalytic term used to describe how unresolved childhood trauma is re-enacted in adulthood. This is discussed more in Chapter 8, "Treatment with the Favored Parent."

Chapter 3

ASSESSMENT PROCEDURES FOR MENTAL HEALTH PROFESSIONALS (CLINICIANS)

> **Learning Objectives:**
> 1. Understand the importance of maintaining neutrality when assessing and working with the family.
> 2. Understand how pertinent legal information and facts about the family of origin can be helpful.
> 3. Be able to detect signs of contact issues.
> 4. Be able to investigate causes of resistance during the therapeutic process.

Clinicians working with post-divorce dynamics face challenges when assessing the causes of children's resistance toward one of their parents. The dynamics in these families can be complex and obscure. Maintaining neutrality while gathering data that informs treatment can be difficult when the children and parents are expressing emotional narratives. Clinicians trained to work with the general population may not be prepared for the level of assessment needed to understand the dynamics operating in these families.

While you may be able to explore some aspects of these dynamics during therapy sessions, it is unrealistic to expect that you could capture a full understanding of the family's situation solely from therapeutic interactions. Mental health professionals providing counseling services to divorcing families are not expected to conduct an assessment like a forensic evaluator would; however, you will need to obtain and review more information than you do with other counseling clients who are not engaged in divorce litigation (Baker et al., 2020; Polak, 2020).

It is essential for you to assess the family dynamics as much as possible so you are not basing your interventions on misperceptions and ultimately causing harm to the family and damaging relationships. A deeper understanding can reveal hidden dynamics operating within the family system and work more effectively toward improving the family's situation (Woodall & Woodall, 2017). If the divorce is relatively new and the family is just now attempting to discover their new normal, it may be easier for you to discern the factors impacting the parent-child relationships. If you come into the case after the behavior patterns have existed for an extended period, it will be more difficult to disentangle the causes. This increasing entrenchment can complicate intervention efforts, make behavioral change more challenging, and warrant a more thorough understanding of the individual and family dynamics (Walters & Friedlander, 2010).

If there is a custody evaluation or another type of forensic assessment being conducted on the family, your understanding of the causes for the parent-child contact issues will likely be enhanced when you review the report. However, it is impractical, and often detrimental, to delay interventions waiting for a full custody evaluation. Many experts recommend initiating family-system based interventions even before an evaluation or court case reaches its conclusion (Deutsch et al., 2020; Greenberg et al., 2019; Greenberg & Schnider, 2020). The rationale behind this approach is that early therapeutic intervention can help reduce the entrenched resist/refuse behaviors and start the process of rebuilding damaged parent-child relationships. This can leave clinicians with limited information, outside of what the client reports, to explain the child's resistance to the parent. This chapter aims to broaden your assessment skills so that you can better understand the underlying dynamics and develop treatment plans that accurately address the origins of the contact issues.

ASSESSMENT RESOURCES FOR CLINICIANS

Pertinent Legal Information

The assessment process should begin with an understanding of the legal orders in place for the family. You will need a basic understanding of what happens in your state when a divorce is filed, the difference between temporary and final orders, the importance of mediated settlement agreements, and the importance of final hearings. This will not only ensure that you are following the legal orders but also help you provide the appropriate emotional support and guidance at each stage.

You will also need to understand the different types of custody (joint, sole, possessory, etc.) and how the child's time is split between the parties. Likewise, a knowledge of legal restrictions such as restraining orders, supervised visitation, and other court orders on the case is essential for ensuring that therapeutic advice does not conflict with legal requirements. Protective orders between the parents often require that they maintain a specific distance from one another and not have any electronic communication. In this case, the therapist would be violating the protective order if they sent out an email addressed to both parents and/or scheduled back-to-back sessions where the parents crossed paths in the office.

It is necessary to request a copy of any existing court orders to determine the other parent's visitation and custody rights and to determine if consent from the other parent is needed for their child to engage in therapy. If the preferred parent does not want you to contact the other parent, that should serve as a red flag for you. It could be that there are true issues with the other parent interfering with therapy, or it could be that the preferred parent wants to make sure that you do not hear a competing perspective on the family situation.

Clinicians should NEVER advise a family member to disobey the court order. For instance, just because the child says that they would like to change the schedule, the therapist should not advise the parents that changing the schedule would be good for the child. The therapist can make the child's wishes known but should avoid making any recommendations about the schedule. Unfortunately, many clinicians make this mistake and receive valid board complaints for doing so. These cases can get very complex, and it is important that you continually evaluate whether you are *staying in your lane* as a clinician. This is addressed in more detail in the book's closing chapter on professional liability.

It is also essential to understand the roles of the various court-appointed child advocates. Every state may have different titles and duties for each role, but if you understand the role of a guardian ad litem, amicus attorney, attorney ad litem, and other court-appointed professionals, you may be able to collaborate more effectively with these professionals.

Collateral Consults

Speaking with other professionals about the family member(s) you are treating is an excellent way to gather data you might not otherwise know. When reviewing the legal orders for the family, you can make note of the other professionals who have been appointed to the case. You should ensure that the parents sign HIPAA releases for you to speak to the court-appointed professionals named in the order and any other professionals with whom the family is working (e.g., family therapists, individual therapists, psychiatrists, etc.).

These professionals will likely have a perspective on the family or on a member of the family that informs your assessment. They may have been working with the family before the separation occurred and be able to provide pre-separation/divorce information about the family dynamics. The quality of the parent-child relationships before separation can be a critical assessment fact when trying to understand contact refusal issues (Baker, 2018; Morrison and Ring, 2021).

If there is a GAL or custody evaluator appointed to the case, they are required to review all pertinent information (e.g., emails, texts, phone recordings, etc.), interview all members of the family, talk to extended family members, consult with educators and childcare providers, among other things. Therefore, their understanding of the family dynamics is informed by multiple sources of information that you, as a therapist, would not have access to nor have the time to review.

Custody evaluators or forensic psychologists may also conduct personality and projective testing on the parents and/or the child, such as the Minnesota Multiphasic Personality Inventory (MMPI-II); the Personality Assessment Inventory (PAI); Milan Clinical Multi-Axial Inventory (MCMI); and the Rorschach. These tests are only available to mental health providers with certain credentials. Counselors, psychotherapists, and licensed clinical social workers do not generally use these measurements as part of a normal therapeutic practice. However, the information resulting from these testing instruments can help determine the treatment needs of the client. Clinicians can ask the client for a copy of the report if it has already been completed or they can obtain a HIPAA release and consult with the evaluator.

Testing Instruments

While it may not be feasible for therapeutic professionals to conduct extensive testing, it is possible to conduct some preliminary screening assessments that can provide useful baseline information about clients. Much of the literature suggests that the initial phase of therapy should involve the therapist undertaking a variety of screening activities to understand the overall dynamics within the family better, especially whether estrangement and/or alienation is involved. One program, Families in Transition, involves an initial comprehensive assessment phase of therapy that is focused on learning about each parent and the child, understanding the needs and worries of the parents, and figuring out if there's any risk for the child when they start reconnecting with the rejected parent (Freeman et al., 2004). Options for initial assessments are:

1. **The Parental Acceptance Rejection Questionnaire** (PARQ) (Rohner, 2008).
   The PARQ is a 60-item questionnaire given to children that measures a child's attitudes toward their parents. It was originally developed to inform theoretical understanding of how parental acceptance and rejection affect personality development and psychological adjustment. It has also been used in custody evaluations and, more recently, in parental alienation assessments. In a study looking at the differences in PARQ scores between children who were neglected and children that were alienated, researchers found that children from intact families had similar rejection scores for each parent, neglected children had a slightly elevated rejection score for the parent who had been abusive, and alienated children had a substantially elevated rejection score for the parent with who they were irrationally rejecting (Bernet et al., 2020). This supported the "lack of ambivalence" characteristic found in alienated children and provided support that alienated children reject a parent at higher level than abused children. (See the diagram below). The PARQ can be ordered from Rohner Research Publications at www.rohnerresearchpublications.com.

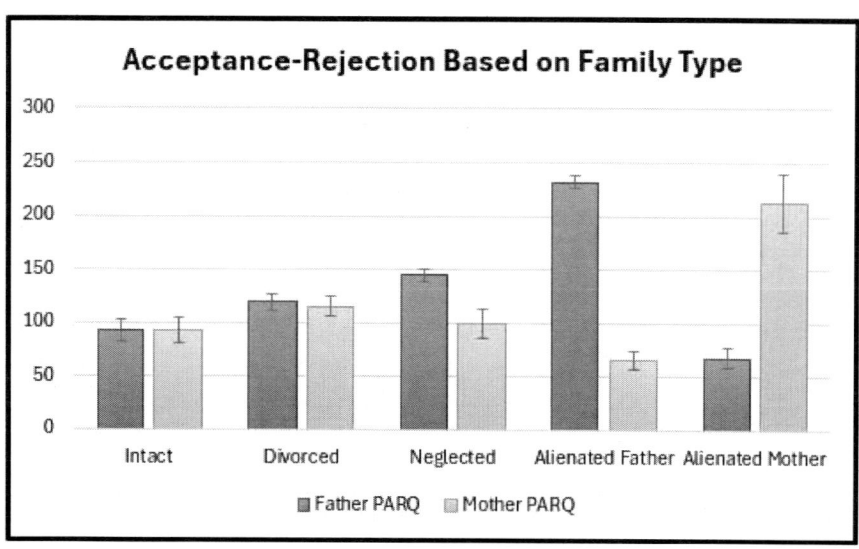

Note: Adapted from "An Objective measure of Splitting in Parental Alienation: The Parental Acceptance-Rejection Questionnaire" by W. Bernet, N. Gregory, K. M. Reay, and R. P. Rohner, 2018, Journal of Forensic Science, 63(3), p. 178 (Doi: 10.1111/1556-4029.13625). Copyright 2018 by Wiley Online Library.

2. **The Beck Depression Inventory** (BDI-II) (Beck et al., 1996).
   The BDI is a 21-item self-report questionnaire that measures symptoms of depression. It is used as a diagnostic tool to help clinicians identify the level of treatment the client may need. The instrument can be used with clients ages 13 to 80. The questions have multiplechoice answers, and it takes about 10 minutes to complete. The BDI has been tested internationally across populations and found to be reliable and valid. The instrument can be purchased through Pearson Assessments at www.pearsonassessments.com.
3. **The Beck Anxiety Inventory** (BAI) (Beck et al., 1988).
   The BAI is a 21-item self-report inventory that measures anxiety levels in adolescents and adults. Each item is a physical symptom, emotional state, or fearful experience, such as a racing heart, nervousness, or fear of losing control. The client rates the level at which they experience the item (not at all, mildly, moderately, or severely). The instrument can be ordered from Pearson Assessments.
4. **Parenting Stress Index** (PSI) (Abidin, 1985).
   The PSI is given to parents and assesses the level of stress the parent experiences in three domains of parenting: (1) child

characteristics, (2) parent characteristics, and (3) situational/demographic life stress. It is used as a screening tool to identify parenting issues that may lead to behavior problems in the child or parent. It can be given in long form (120 items) and takes about 20 minutes, or in short form (PSI-4-SF) (36 items), which only takes about 10 minutes to complete. The long form has been translated into 28 languages and has been shown to be reliable and valid across diverse populations. To order this instrument, contact PAR at www.parinc.com or 1-800-331-8378.

Historical Timelines

It can be helpful to have the child and each parent provide a timeline of events from their individual perspectives that led to contact refusal. This can be done verbally in conversation with the therapist or independently in a written format. When there is complete contact refusal, there is usually the "straw that broke the camel's back" or the defining moment where the child refuses contact with the parent. Delineating the events that led up to that moment can increase your understanding of the behaviors that contributed to the contact refusal and allow you to better address those behaviors with the child and/or the parents.

The parent with whom the child is aligned may attempt to use those behaviors to undermine the therapeutic process or the therapeutic relationship between you and the child, further complicating the situation and impeding the child's progress. Clinicians should stay alert to information in the timelines that describes the power dynamics within the family (e.g., who holds more influence; who is more passive; does the more powerful parent influence the children, and if so, how; are differing opinions allowed and expressed; has a child been elevated to a parental role, if so, which parent allowed/encouraged that) and use that information to begin to realign the family in a healthier way (Woodall & Woodall, 2017).

Family of Origin Information

Woodall (2017) addresses the idea of how patterns of justified or unjustified estrangement in the history of either or both parents may have been passed down through generations. These behaviors might have been internalized as standard conduct within the family.

Patterns of estrangement may originate from previous generations and normalize within the family over time. They may manifest as familial habits, traditions, or behavioral codes that shape how family members interact with one another.

The current separation and divorce can trigger unconscious behavioral patterns and emotions related to childhood experiences and emerge within the current family system. The parent may or may not be aware of how these patterns contribute to their current behaviors. Therapists can assess the parent's level of consciousness regarding these patterns by drawing connections between childhood experiences and current feelings and behaviors. When increased awareness and insight lead to a change in behavior, clinicians gain information that the parent did not understand how they were negatively influencing the child and reenacting old relationship traumas. When the parent is not able to internalize the similarities between their own childhood experiences and their current behaviors, clinicians gain information that the parent's capacity for insight and, therefore, change may be limited (Woodall, 2017).

Transitions and Exchanges

As a clinician, you can easily gain information about the child's transitions between the parents. This is valuable information when ascertaining the causes and concerns about parent-child contact issues. When children are in an intact family, they naturally form attachments to the adult figures in their lives who are responsive to their needs. Woodall and Woodall (2017) discuss the construct of the "transition bridge" to describe the emotional and psychological tasks a child must navigate to protect attachment relationships when there is a family separation. The model highlights the importance of helping the child manage difficult emotions, adapt to the changing family dynamics, and preserve the attachments with both parents. As they go from one home to the next, there are steps the parents can take that will ease the child's transition to the other home.

Most working parents know how a young child may transition from their arms to that of a caregiver while the parent goes to work. If the parent lingers and anxiously awaits the transition, the child may become anxious about going to the other caregiver, too. On the other hand, if the parent is positive about the transition, the child will, in time, adjust quickly to it.

Similar dynamics can often be seen when a child is having difficulty transitioning from Parent A to Parent B; that is, Parent A may be seen belaboring the transition with messages such as, "You only have to be there for three sleeps," and "I am going to miss you so much—are you going to miss me?" and "Just remember to pray every time you are scared." These messages can create emotions of fear about missing out on things and/or going to the other parent's home. If one parent talks about how the child does not want to go to the other parent's house, the behaviors of the complaining parent can create more anxiety for the child and make it difficult for that child to transition to the other home.

Signs of Contact Issues in the Therapy Room.

A clinician who understands the issues that often arise in homes affected by divorce will start to unravel and identify any dysfunctional dynamics that might be present. When the primary issue involves problems with parent-child contact, an informed practitioner will promptly start differentiating the case. This involves identifying the specific factors and situations that contribute to the child's refusal or resistance to interact with one parent.

However, there are also cases where the issues related to parent-child contact are not immediately apparent. These problems might start to emerge as the therapist works more closely with the family and delves deeper into their dynamics and interactions. Let's explore some ways you might start seeing these parent-child contact issues come to light during your work with the family.

Child as Client

A child whose parents are divorcing can be brought to your office for a wide range of problems. These include, but are not limited to, concerns related to behavior, academic performance, depression, anxiety, diminished self-confidence, and difficulties with interpersonal relationships. Each of these may negatively impact the child's overall functioning. On occasion, the exhibited behaviors of the child may be an outward manifestation of the underlying familial dysfunction.

Therefore, psychotherapists specializing in working with children must adopt a more systems-level perspective. This allows them to appreciate the factors potentially contributing to the challenges faced by the child. By engaging in a more thorough and dynamic exploration of the child's environment, you can more effectively address the multifaceted nature of their difficulties, leading to more sustainable solutions.

When the child comes from a family context of divorce, the treatment planning to address emotional and behavioral concerns may be complicated by needing to understand the dynamics in both households. Regrettably, it is common for therapists to engage with only one of the parents. While this may seem like an efficient course, it can be classified as negligent and potentially undermine the validity of the treatment planning. Even in instances where one parent possesses the legal right to initiate therapy without the express consent of the other parent, it remains highly beneficial for the clinician to reach out to the other parent. This approach provides a broader and more holistic understanding of the child's circumstances, thereby facilitating more effective therapeutic interventions (Baker et al., 2020).

In some cases, both parents want the child in therapy and are concerned about the child resisting or refusing contact with a parent. These resist/refuse behaviors may arise due to numerous factors including but not limited to high-conflict divorces, parental alienation, the child's reaction to the changes surrounding the divorce, or negative perceptions about the noncustodial parent (Johnston et al., 2005; see Chapter 2 for more discussion). Clinicians need to remain cognizant of their role and be aware that they are likely not privy to enough information to know the reasons for the resistance in the child immediately.

The clinician mustn't automatically determine whether the child's rationale is justified or unjustified. In fact, the therapist should aim to investigate these issues further during the intake process with both parents and the therapy sessions with the child. They might want to learn more about the child's feelings and experiences, as this could give them more insight into why the child is resisting contact with their parent (Smith, 2016).

Parents as Clients

A clinician may encounter issues related to parent-child contact when two divorced parents seek help to improve their co-parenting skills. One parent might express concerns about the living conditions or atmosphere at the other parent's house and how it affects their child.

In these instances, the mental health professional should investigate the truth behind these claims before trying to resolve the issues.

There are instances where the parent raising these concerns might have legitimate worries about their child's well-being in the other parent's house. On the other hand, these concerns might stem from differences in parenting styles. If that is the case, the concerned parent might need to accept that the other parent has a different way of parenting and that it is okay for both parents to approach raising their child differently.

Furthermore, a clinician should help the parents understand if they are unintentionally putting their child in a difficult position by making them feel like they must choose between their parents. The more a child feels caught in the middle of their parents' issues, the more challenging it can become for them to adjust to moving back and forth between two households (Bernet et al., 2016). The parents should not be complaining in front of the child about how the other parent is running the household, even if that parent feels they are just validating the child's frustrations. The clinician's role is to help the parents navigate these issues, find solutions that prioritize the child's well-being, and minimize emotional stress.

Reactions to Intervention

When the authors were learning to work with these families, they relied heavily on the training developed by Karen and Nick Woodall, who taught that "intervention informs assessment." This wisdom has proven to be true repeatedly over the years. It refers to new information that can be revealed about a client's willingness to make changes when the clinician asks the client to do something different to improve the parent-child relationship problem.

As stated previously, parents engaged in custody litigation often have personal and legal agendas that influence their presentation to mental health professionals. The following vignette provides an example of this dynamic works.

Case Vignette: Mr. Howard and Mia

Mr. Howard had been separated from his wife for six months. He had three children and the oldest daughter, Mia, refused to see her mother on the agreed parenting time schedule. Mia had not seen her mother in the six months since the separation.

> A guardian ad litem (GAL) was appointed to conduct an assessment to determine the causes for Mia's refusal to see her mother and an individual therapist was appointed to work with Mia. Mr. Howard did not believe Mia should have to see her mother if she did not want to and believed that Mia had good reason not to adhere to the parenting time schedule. He believed that Mia's mother engaged in overly harsh parenting practices that warranted Mia's resistance.
>
> Mr. Howard's attorney advised him that he should NOT share his support of Mia's refusal with the GAL or the therapist because they may see him as obstructing the parent-child relationship. Mr. Howard adhered to his attorney's advice and told the GAL and the therapist that he would do whatever was necessary to support Mia's relationship with her mother.

In this case example, the father's genuine desire was to limit the mother's access to the child after the divorce, but his statements to the professionals were the opposite. A clinician would only see the father's true level of resistance by asking the father to do something (e.g., tell Mia she needs to go to her mother's, enforce the parenting time schedule, tell Mia positive things about her mother, etc.). The father, in this scenario, found it impossible to do any of these things and became angry at the GAL for recommending parenting time for Mia and her mother and angry at the therapist for supporting the recommendations. Hence, the intervention (i.e., asking dad to support or enforce Mia's time with mom) informed the assessment of the factors contributing to Mia's resistance.

Another example where the parent's interference in the child's relationship with the other parent was more obvious initially but then became more covert after therapeutic intervention is provided in the following case vignette.

Case Vignette: Larry and Leah

> Larry and Leah were newly separated. They agreed to put their child Beau into individual therapy. Leah did not want a divorce and was grieving. She and Beau had always been extremely close because she had been a stay-at-home mom and had been involved in every facet of his life. Larry and Beau were also close, but Larry was the family's provider and had been required to travel often for work. Beau expressed his concern about his mother to his therapist. She often cried at night because she missed his dad and was afraid they would not have enough money. Beau would attempt to comfort her. Beau told his therapist that he did not want to see his father because he was mad at his dad for hurting his mother and for leaving her without money

to take care of them.

    The therapist asked to speak to Leah individually and told her that she needed to stop confiding in Beau because it was causing emotional harm to Beau and interfering with his positive feelings for his father. Leah expressed gratitude to the therapist, stating that she wanted to learn more about protecting Beau and his relationship with his father. The therapist believed that Leah was genuine and would stop sharing her emotions with Beau. Beau stopped expressing concern about his mother in therapy; however, he also stopped engaging in therapeutic activities and started expressing a dislike for therapy.

    Additionally, the therapist spoke with the GAL on the case and discovered that Beau's resistance to his father had increased and that Beau was telling teachers that his dad was mistreating him. Beau was not discussing these things with his therapist. The therapist's treatment changed to a more non-directive approach until the forensic evaluators could complete their full assessment. This allowed Beau to relax in therapy and continue to use therapy to process emotions.

In this case scenario, the intervention appeared to work because the mother appeared receptive to the feedback, and the child quit discussing his negativity about the father. Though, it only served to educate the mother and son that they should not speak about their conversations to the therapist. While this was not helpful to the therapeutic process, it did help to inform the forensic assessment and clarified the extent to which the mother would go to interfere in the child's relationship with his father. It also provided information about the mother's willingness to manipulate others to get what she wanted.

In summary, the way family members respond to therapeutic intervention can provide valuable observations into the dynamics influencing parent-child relationships. Their reactions can clarify their levels of genuine interest in improving relationships (Woodall & Woodall, 2017). Clinicians must be willing to adjust their clinical conclusions as new information is presented.

Neutrality/Bias

Maintaining neutrality and monitoring bias involves being ready to revise your initial assumptions if new information emerges that leads to a different conclusion. One of the key challenges that evaluators and therapists must navigate is the risk of bias, both in the sources of information they are analyzing and within their own interpretations

(Lillenfeld & Bowes, 2018).

Confirmation bias is a common pitfall that can profoundly influence one's fairness. It refers to the tendency to search for, interpret, favor, and recall information in a way that confirms one's preexisting beliefs or hypotheses. In the context of a family assessment by a clinician, this bias might manifest as the therapist selectively attending to information that aligns with their initial assumptions about the family's dynamics and ignoring or minimizing conflicting evidence. The following vignette demonstrates how confirmation bias can develop and impede therapeutic progress.

Case Vignette: Isabel

Isabel was an eleven-year-old girl who had made sexual abuse allegations about her father. She came in with her mom, who was very domineering in the first session and answered the questions presented to Isabel. It was evident that Isabel had signs of trauma, and her medical history gave her a diagnosis of irritable bowel syndrome that her doctor linked to the sexual abuse she experienced. When Isabel came into the clinician's office and talked about her family, she avoided talking about her dad altogether. When doing artwork representing her family, she did not include her dad. The clinician at one point gently prodded about her dad, and Isabel, who usually had a quiet demeanor, snapped at the clinician, saying she never wanted to talk or hear about him again because he had sexually abused her.

A Guardian ad Litem was investigating the case and shared with the clinician that some were questioning the validity of the sexual abuse allegations. The GAL pointed out to Isabel's therapist that the dad had passed a polygraph test, and Isabel's therapist correctly pointed out that polygraphs were not admissible in court. The dad was also seeing his own mental health professional, who did not believe that he had sexually abused his daughter. Isabel's individual clinician did not believe that dad's clinician would have any way to know whether his client was innocent or guilty as he had not seen the traumatic responses evident in Isabel. The clinician quickly dismissed any evidence that did not match what was being observed in her office. When Isabel's clinician was called to testify in court, she testified that it was evident that Isabel had faced some sexual trauma and she was going to continue to need some trauma therapy. The clinician testified that in no way should Isabel ever be asked to see her father, not even in a therapeutic setting.

Months later, after a more thorough investigation was completed, it was found that her father, in fact, did not abuse her. Instead, her mom had coached her to make these allegations and was telling her what to say in therapy and making sure that Isabel kept the story straight. The court ordered that Isabel go to her father with her aunt as a supervisor and not have contact with her mother for an extended period. Isabel's clinician was horrified that they would put a child with her abuser, even if it was with supervision. When told she was not going to see her mom for a long time and she was instead going to be with her dad and aunt, Isabel was immediately relieved and described all the things her mom did to make her say things about her dad, including having to record therapy sessions and being chastised for not being convincing enough in those sessions about being sexually abused. She felt bad that she had lied to her therapist, but she felt like she had to.

Unfortunately, this kind of scenario can easily happen in these cases, especially if a clinician is not well-trained in resist-refuse dynamics. The individual therapist refused even to consider some of the concerns of the GAL even though the therapist knew the guardian had reviewed much more information about the case. To avoid this bias, mental health professionals must consciously strive for objectivity, continually challenging their own assumptions and earnestly trying to keep an open hypothesis. Awareness of confirmation bias is the first step to mitigating its effects, but continuous efforts to remain neutral are required to ensure a balanced, fair, and accurate evaluation (Lillenfeld & Bowes, 2018).

Areas of Investigation for Causes of Resistance

It is crucial to consider the various hypotheses that could explain the child's behavior and/or emotional symptoms. Some potential causes might be perfectly reasonable, while others might indicate an issue to be remedied. Although one parent may provide their perspective or interpretation of the situation, it is vital for the evaluator to form their own conclusions. These should be based on an unbiased review of all the data gathered, not just the narrative presented by one or both parents, or even the child's perspective (Freeman, 2004).

If the primary concern is the child's refusal of contact with one parent, clinicians must consider all the potential causes. These may include normal developmental preferences, such as a natural affinity for one parent over the other, or reactions to specific circumstances related to the divorce. Other possibilities include estrangement resulting from a parent's neglectful or abusive behavior, parental alienation, or a situation where the child is either excessively worried or stubbornly resistant. The child might also be attempting to avoid conflict, leading to their refusal of contact (Bernet, 2006; Johnston, 2005). Each of these potential reasons can contribute to the child's behavior in different ways. The previous chapter offers a more thorough examination of these reasons, providing an in-depth exploration of how they might influence a child's interactions with their parents after a divorce or separation.

To summarize, as a clinician, you likely will not have access to the full picture unless you have access to a forensic evaluation that has been completed on the family, so it is important that you are even-handed as you work with the family and attempt to discover the underlying currents that may be impacting the family. Practically speaking, when your client is the child, neutrality will entail having as equal time as you can with each parent, attempting to have each parent take turns bringing the child in for therapy, and ensuring that you are able to understand each parent's perspective. Even if you find yourself agreeing with one parent more, it is important that you continue to have empathy for the other parent's position. Clinicians should recognize the limitations of the information they depend on and stay open-minded about anything that challenges their beliefs about the family (Fidler & Bala, 2020).

A thorough assessment of family dynamics can significantly aid in identifying and selecting appropriate interventions to address all the issues that may be co-occurring. Once these elements have been identified, individualized interventions can be tailored to each specific issue. If a forensic assessment is being conducted on the family, clinicians can use the evaluation to inform their treatment planning. This focused approach helps ensure that each concern is addressed in the most effective manner in treatment planning to facilitate overall resolution (Friedlander & Walters, 2010).

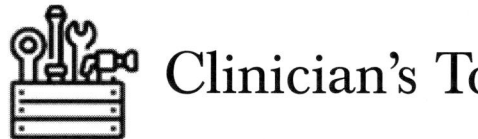 Clinician's Toolbox

- ✗ Questions you may want to ask yourself when working with the family:
- ✗ Normal developmental preferences:
    - Is the child more aligned with the parent with shared interests?
    - Is the child more aligned with the parent of the same gender?
    - Is the child younger and more aligned with the primary

caregiver?
- Does the favored parent promote more engagement with the child's friends?
- Does the favored parent support the child's activities more than the other parent?
- Does the less preferred parent have significant parenting skills/deficits (less nurturing, less understanding, or less engaged with the child in general)?

✗ Reactions to circumstances of divorce:
- Is the child hurt by one parent's reason for leaving the family?
- Did one parent leave in a manner that was hurtful to the child?
- Does the child feel sorry for the preferred parent?
- Does the child disapprove of the other parent's actions?

✗ Avoiding Loyalty Conflict:
- Is the child feeling pressure to take sides in parental disagreements?
- Is the child well aware of the parents' dislike for each other?

✗ Characteristics of the Child:
- Is the child predisposed to depression or anxiety?
- Does the child have difficulty with change?

✗ Enmeshment:
- Does the child and/or favored parent use the word "we" when describing personal experiences, preferences, or opinions?
- Do the parent and the favored parent seem very close?
- Does the child struggle with age-appropriate independence?
- Does the child sit unusually close to the preferred parent in session?

✗ Parental Alienation-intentional or unintentional:
- Does the child have any of the above information (reason for leaving the family, knowledge of the court process, knowledge of parental conflict) filtered through the perspective of the favored parent?
- Does the favored parent purposefully schedule activities on the other parent's time to make it appear that the other parent is not supportive of activities?
- Does the preferred parent exhibit anxiety when the child is

transitioning to the other parent's home? Examples include letting the child know how much they will miss the child, praying for the child before going, and letting the child know how many days they "have to be" with the other parent.
- Does the child exhibit many or all of the eight manifestations?
- Are you able to observe any alienating strategies on the part of the favored parent?

Chapter 4

CASES INVOLVING ABUSE ALLEGATIONS: DIFFERENTIATING BETWEEN ESTRANGEMENT AND PARENTAL ALIENATION

> **Learning Objectives:**
> 1. Understand the differences between the characteristics of an abused child and the characteristics of an alienated child.
> 2. Understand the Five Factor Model of Parental Alienation.
> 3. Understand the collateral information that may be relevant when preparing treatment plans for children and/or families when abuse allegations have been made.
> 4. Understand the differences in reunification treatment for a child who has been abused and a child affected by parental alienation.

Mental health professionals working with parent-child contact issues are frequently faced with situations where the child's reasons for wanting no contact or relationship with a parent include allegations of abuse. In many cases, the therapeutic work with the family begins before an evaluation, investigation, or court hearing has determined whether the allegations are credible. Individual and/or family therapy may have been agreed to by the parents, by the attorneys, or recommended by the guardian ad litem, which can create a treatment planning challenge since the approach to resolving the issue depends on whether the allegations are substantiated or not.

During the initial appointments, the child may express hatred or fear for one parent and adamantly refuse to ever see the parent again. The child's narrative may be highly emotional and include allegations of alarming behavior by the parent. If the rejected parent acknowledges abusive behavior, your approach to reunification is clear and would follow a child protection approach to include parenting education, acknowledgment and apology to the child, and trust-building exercises. When child protection agencies find reason to believe that abuse has occurred, they usually implement a safety plan that includes rehabilitation for the abusive parent and safety measures for the child. Mental health professionals working with the family have access to these treatment plans.

However, when the assessment is incomplete or inconclusive, clinicians may find themselves going back and forth between the child's accusations and strong resistance and the rejected parent's grief and descriptions of themselves as a good enough parent. The parent whom the child favors reports a similar narrative to the child's, and the parent whom the child is refusing has a opposite storyline that offers genuine examples of loving, fun, and warm interactions with the child. It would not be therapeutic to force a client who has been abused to face their abuser until they are ready. However, if the child is alienated and professing a false or extremely exaggerated narrative, it does not support their psychological health to reinforce their narrative which developed as a response to loyalty binds, parental pressure, psychological manipulation, and/or alienating behaviors from others who do not want the child to have a relationship with the parent.

The child's voice is always an important consideration, except when their voice is not their own and their feelings about a parent are the result of pressure and manipulation. Clinicians working with the child may be asked what the child has reported as their preference and the child's reasons for wanting that. The veracity of the child's statements and the extent to which a parent or older sibling may have influenced their preference should be considered.

Allegations of abuse by the child or the parent are found in approximately a third to a half of contested custody cases involving allegations of parental alienation (Harman & Lorandos, 2020). These allegations should always be taken seriously by the clinician and should be reported if they are not already under investigation. Clinicians working with this population should understand the basic protocols of best practices for documenting and interviewing children who make abuse outcries; however, forensic interviewing should be left to a forensic expert.

Research on child suggestibility blossomed in the late 1980's and 1990's as reports of child abuse increased dramatically. In 1979, there were 669,000 reports of child abuse. By 1990, that number had increased to two million (Myers, 2011). Professionals became somewhat polarized as they grappled with the accuracy of children's reports. On one side of the issue, professionals were saying that a child's outcry should always be believed, and on the other side of the issue, professionals were saying children's memories are malleable and their statements were easily influenced by others. This led to an increase in social science research which revealed the extent to which a child's memory could be influenced by an interviewer, other adults, and other children. Leading questions and repetitive questioning were found to illicit ever-changing and increasingly bizarre memories from children (Ceci & Bruck, 1993; Loftus, 1993).

Two high-profile cases where this research was applicable involved childcare centers. *Margaret Kelly Michaels vs. New Jersey* (1985) and *The People vs. Buckey* (1983). Kelly Michaels, Raymond Buckey, and Virginia Buckey were initially found guilty of multiple counts of child sexual abuse and imprisoned for several years before being exonerated after the interviewing techniques used by law enforcement and mental health professionals were found to lead and, at times, pressure the children to make statements that they thought the interviewers wanted to hear. What professionals learned from these cases and the research of that time still guide best practices today when interviewing children (Baker & Eichler, 2023). For those interested in more information on the interviewing and investigative processes found to skew children's reports of abuse, HBO made a movie based on the Buckey case entitled "Indictment: The McMartin Trial" (Schneider, 1995).

In child custody cases, false allegations of abuse occur more frequently than in the normal population. Researchers have found that a third to one-half of sexual abuse allegations in custody litigation were unsubstantiated. Less than 10% of the unsubstantiated sexual abuse allegations were found to be purposeful in their intent to lie about the actions of the accused person (Trocmé & Bala, 2005). Blush and Ross (1987) were one of the first to review the nature of child sexual abuse allegations in relation to custody and visitation. They emphasized the importance of carefully reviewing the legal history of a case, evaluating sequence, escalation, and timing factors.

Kuehnle and Kirkpatrick (2005) consider child sexual abuse in high-conflict custody cases utilizing the Conceptual Framework Hypothesis. With a particular family system, the hypotheses with this framework would be:

1. The child is not a victim of child sexual abuse and is credible but is estranged from the identified parent and has misperceived an innocent or ambiguous interaction.
2. The child is not a victim of child sexual abuse, but the parent is alleging sexual abuse to manipulate the legal system to secure the child to stay with her, giving her all the rights and responsibilities, and effectively ending her and the child's relationship with the accused parent.
3. The child is a victim of child sexual abuse, and these are credible allegations. Relative to these three hypotheses, a critical question in this matter concerns whether the child was a victim of sexual abuse. At this time, there are no standardized instruments that can reliably differentiate child victims of sexual abuse from non-sexually abused children (Kuehnle, 2002).

There is also no cluster of symptoms that reliably demonstrate that a child has been sexually abused. Children who are victims of child sexual abuse have symptoms that vary widely, and some may not exhibit any symptoms at all (Kendall-Tackett et al., 1993). Furthermore, research has not found any statistically significant differences in therapeutic interactions with dolls, sand trays, or drawings (Kuehnle & Connell, 2009). Gratz and Orsillo (2003) performed a comprehensive review of the literature on child sexual abuse. They concluded that there is no ethical way to conclude that sexual abuse has occurred based on the child's behaviors and symptoms after the alleged abuse.

Clinicians should stay alert to the potential of false reporting when working with families in divorce. Most mental health professionals, judges, and parents will believe that any child who makes a sexual abuse allegation must be telling the truth (MacKay, 2014). Making the situation more complex is the fact that many mental health professionals believe they can differentiate true from false sexual abuse allegations, but research has found high error rates among the mental health professionals who do assess for sexual abuse (Herman, 2005; Herman & Freitas, 2010; Bala et al., 2007, Brown, 2003, Johnston et al., 2005, Poole & Lindsay, 1998).

It should not fall to the clinician to determine whether abuse occurred or not. Clinicians are mandatory reporters, not mandatory investigators; however, mental health professionals should understand the components of reliable interviewing techniques to avoid eliciting untrue statements or minimizing legitimate concerns. Association of Family and Conciliation Courts (AFCC) (2011) guideline 3.3 for court-involved therapists states that therapists should maintain current knowledge on "Child interviewing and suggestibility" and on "Children's decision-making ability, including appropriate means of understanding children's abilities and interpreting expressed preferences or opinions" (p. 10).

Details of an event can morph with multiple reiterations of the story. Bruck and Ceci (1995) identified major interviewer flaws during the Wee Care childcare case that led to erroneous conclusions, increased trauma to children, wrongful convictions, and social hysteria. They found that interviewers (1) held preconceived notions that children were abused, which led to an interviewing goal aimed at getting children to admit that they had been abused, (2) neglected to consider alternative hypotheses for the child's statements, (3) used leading questions, (4) used an intimidating tone when the children did not answer a question with an answer that confirmed the interviewer's preconceived belief, and (5) did not follow up on inconsistent statements.

Some parents are intentional in their efforts to interfere with the child's relationship with the other parent, for example, by making unfounded abuse allegations, knowing there is no actual risk to the child. Cases involving malicious allegations, however, occur less frequently than those where the parent, though intentional in their restrictive protective gatekeeping, has a genuine belief that the child is at risk despite the findings of child protection investigation or the family courts that abuse has not occurred (Saini et al., 2020; Fidler & Bala, 2020). To make the most appropriate treatment recommendations for such a family, the strengths and weaknesses of the sexual abuse allegation must be considered as it cannot be determined with complete certainty whether it happened or not.

Research on children who reject a parent during separation and divorce has shown some differences between the rational resistance of an abused child and the irrational resistance of an alienated child (Baker et al., 2012; Baker & Schneiderman, 2015; Baker et al., 2019; Bernet et al., 2019). Caseworkers working with abused children who have been placed in foster care report that most of their clients want to see their abusive parents and look forward to a time when they can be reunited, even when they understand that for their safety, they need to live apart from them (Baker et al., 2019). Bernet and colleagues (2019) found that children who had experienced abuse by a parent had less polarized views of their parents than children who were alienated. Children who were abused tended to cherish positive memories and were more likely to see the good in their abusive parent than children who were irrationally rejecting a parent due to the manipulation or pressure of the favored parent. Baker et al. (2012) found that children referred to a counseling clinic by the court for reunification therapy due to irrational rejection of a parent, as compared to children referred to the clinic for various reasons having to do with high conflict divorce, described their parents in terms of all good and all bad. The favored parents were described as having no faults, while the rejected parents were described as having no positive qualities at all. The children in the reunification group could not remember one positive memory about the rejected parent.

Clinicians can assess the amount of healthy ambivalence in the child's statements about their parents as an indicator for rational versus irrational rejection of a parent during separation and divorce. These unique characteristics may help you weigh the likelihood of whether the resistance the child has toward the parent is caused by abusive parenting or an unhealthy alignment between the child and the favored parent. This is by no means the only variable to assess when deciding whether the rejection of the parent is justified or not. Still, it is one of the most easily observable characteristics in a counseling setting and will help you maintain alternative explanations while other investigations are being completed.

THE FIVE-FACTOR MODEL OF PARENTAL ALIENATION

The Five-Factor Model is a framework for organizing information in cases where a child is rejecting a parent during separation and divorce. It was designed to help differentiate between estrangement (justified rejection) and parental alienation (unjustified rejection). It has been shown to be a reliable and valid tool (Baker, 2018; Morrison &

Ring, 2021). All five factors must be satisfied, with a few exceptions, for the child's resistance to be caused purely by parental alienation. Clinicians working therapeutically with the family will not typically collect enough information to use the model. Still, their understanding of the factors may help them maintain and assess alternative hypotheses regarding parent-child relational issues during separation and divorce.

One criticism of the Five Factor model is that it is a binary tool, requiring an over simplistic yes or no assessment for each factor, not allowing for the complexity of family dynamics to be assessed (Garber & Simon, 2023). The authors have not found the application of the Five-Factor Model to be simplistic or binary. For example, establishing that there was a previous positive relationship between the child and the parent is necessary to satisfy the second factor in the model. To prove that there was a previous positive relationship, the parents must provide evidence to support that claim. Satisfaction of the factor is determined by the weight of the evidence, which usually consists of pictures, texts, videos, mementos and gifts, and collateral reports to name a few. Evidence provided from all these sources would likely satisfy this criterion, whereas one photo album with pictures of the child and parent five years ago likely would not unless the child had been kept from the parent for the last five years. A simplistic "yes or no" requirement to satisfy this factor would not consider the amount of evidence, the type of evidence, or the number of various sources providing evidence. An evaluator may find that the parental involvement was excessive and controlling and explain that although parental involvement was present, it did not represent a healthy and positive relationship.

Factor One

Factor one is the threshold factor for alienation to be considered and states that the child must be resisting a relationship with one parent. Contact resistance and refusal can manifest for many reasons during divorce and separation. This model can be used as part of an evaluation to determine if the refusal is justified or unjustified. Resistance to a parent can occur at varying levels ranging from mild to severe, where milder levels are characterized by continued contact between the parent and child and severe levels usually include a refusal to have any contact with the parent. In some situations, a child can be classified as severely alienated even though they are still transitioning between two homes according to the court-ordered schedule. Their behavior at the rejected parent's home is withdrawn, hostile, and/or extremely disrespectful. In some cases, the child will stay in their room for the entire weekend and refuse to interact with any family member.

Factor Two

Factor two requires the rejected parent and child to have a prior positive relationship. When the child resists contact with a parent, they may say that they never liked the parent. The favored parent may also report that the child and the rejected parent never got along and never spent any quality time together. In this scenario, it would be understandable if a child resists spending time with the parent. This factor is assessed by asking for the rejected parent to show you photos, videos, and other tokens of affection or love from the child such as cards, school drawings, and arts and crafts projects. Speaking to extended family members, teachers, and coaches is another way to verify whether a parent was involved with the child and assess the quality of the interactions before the separation or divorce.

It is important to determine when the child's resistance to the parent began. Unhealthy alignment between the child and the favored parent could have started before the separation occurred. If the rejected parent reports that they noticed the child withdrawing a year prior to the separation, the information collected regarding this factor should predate the initial distancing and withdrawal of the child. One exception to this factor is when the parent was not allowed contact with the child from a very early age, eliminating any chance of building a close relationship. For instance, if a parent takes the child shortly after birth and moves to another state and does not allow contact between the child and the other parent, the lack of a prior positive relationship was not because of parenting failures on the part of the rejected parent.

This factor does not require that a parent be a perfect parent. There are no perfect parents. Children build strong attachments to flawed parents all the time. This factor only requires that the parent not be so "incompetent or ineffective or uninvolved that there was no prior attachment" (Baker, 2018, p. 3). "The relevant question is not whether this parent is perfect. It is whether the parent has engaged normative parenting which includes a wide array of parenting styles and behaviors" (Baker, 2020, p. 210).

A common reaction by mental health professionals when dealing with a litany of reasons from the child as to why they do not want to have a relationship with their parent, is to put all their focus on the parent the child is complaining about. Clinicians can ask themselves why these things were not a reason for rejection earlier. Additionally, the favored parent has probably made as many mistakes as the rejected parent. Yet, the child is not refusing contact with them or even acknowledging that the favored parent has ever let them down or disappointed them. In more severe cases of parental alienation, the child's requirements for good enough parenting become hyper-focused on one parent while holding the favored parent to few, if any, standards. This type of polarization should be a red flag for clinicians that the resistance to the parent may be caused by the alienating behaviors of the favored parent.

Factor Three

Factor three requires that there be an absence of abuse by the rejected parent. When abuse allegations have been proven, the child's resistance to the parent is a normal and expected response. As Gardner (1998) stated in his early writings on alienation, "I am referring here to those who are truly innocent of any behavior that warrants the degree of victimization visited upon them by their children" (p. 209).

A characteristic of high-conflict divorce is the involvement of child protective agencies. When a parent or child reports that their reason for not wanting a relationship with one parent is due to abuse, the therapist should inquire about the status of the investigation and request any documents associated with the case. In Texas, the full CPS investigation report is only released by subpoena, so it is difficult to know the details collected in the interviews conducted by the CPS investigator.

One of the lawyers can request the full investigation report, or clinicians can request that parents sign a release and provide the name and contact information of the investigator. Families receive a letter stating whether the agency found cause to believe; however, this provides no information about who was interviewed and what the interviewee said about the situation. A child's report to an interviewer at the time of the incident could be valuable information to consider when the child is making statements about the incident in therapy. Likewise, a parent's description of the event at the time of the incident may also be significant as they relay information in their parent consultation or intake sessions.

If another formal assessment occurs while therapy is taking place, the evaluator conducting the assessment will most likely review the full reports from child protection agencies and include any substantial information in their report. In this case, the clinician would not necessarily need to request the investigation report but should remain mindful that until the evaluator's report is released, a significant amount of information is lacking in their conceptualization of the case.

When abuse is confirmed, the child's rejection of the parent cannot be explained entirely by alienation. Behaviors by the favored parent that could be considered alienating, such as limiting time, are protective when the other parent has abused the child. Abuse findings rule out the possibility of alienation as the sole cause of the rejection, and the therapist's treatment plan will need to include strategies for reunification that address the abuse as opposed to reunification techniques used for parental alienation.

Reunification treatment for parental alienation involves working with distorted memories and cognition errors and provides the child with opportunities to experience the parent and engage in activities with the parent that help the child return to their original attachment with the parent (Warshak, 2018). Reunification for abuse situations provides the abusive parent with education on appropriate discipline, behavior management, and anger management and allows the child a safe place to process the experience and their emotions associated with the abuse. It often includes the parent writing a letter to the child acknowledging the abuse and apologizing. This process will not resolve the resistance of a child who is affected by parental alienation.

For example, one of the authors consulted with child protection professionals on a case where the child was refusing contact with the father. The Department of Health and Family Services found the children's allegations about their father's abusive behavior to be credible, even though there was no physical evidence to support their claims. The children refused to see the father and his extended family, with whom they had spent summers and holidays for most of their lives. The father and the children were asked to attend family therapy with a domestic violence counselor for reunification. The CPS professional did not understand why their usual method of reunification was not working (i.e., acknowledging the child's feelings, and writing a letter of apology). The case worker stated that this process had worked with children who were abused much more severely than the allegations reported in this case. This author reviewed all the documentation in the CPS file, all the documentation related to ten years of custody litigation, interviewed all the family members and found that it was more likely that the children were coached to make the allegations of abuse (parental alienation) than it was that they experienced physical abuse by the father. Therefore, the treatment protocol that was being used for children who have suffered bona fide abuse did not match the treatment needs of these children who were rejecting their father because of their mother's manipulations, not because their father was abusive. The therapist was changed to one who knew how to address parental alienation. The mother was ordered to participate in parenting education to learn how her behavior negatively impacted the children's relationship with their father. The children's time was restored with the father, and the children's resistance decreased.

A counterintuitive aspect of parental alienation is that the more adamantly the child refuses to have a relationship with the parent, the more likely the child's rejection may be caused by alienating behaviors. The phrase "bonded to the abuser" refers to a dynamic where children assume the responsibility for abuse rather than holding their parent accountable. It is rare that a child refuses all contact with a parent, even when there has been abuse and neglect. Adults who were abused as children reported wanting to maintain their relationship with the abusive parent and loving them (Baker & Schneiderman, 2015).

In a survey of 338 mental health providers who worked with moderately and severely abused children, clinicians reported that their clients were more likely to engage in behaviors that maintained their attachments with their abusive caregivers (expressing care about the parent, staying in touch with the caregiver's family, downplaying the harm, wanting a better relationship, etc.) than engage in behaviors that might disrupt the relationship (refusal to have a relationship, being rude or disrespectful to the parent, being uncaring about the parent's feelings, etc.) (Baker et al., 2019). Research studies on attachment theory have also found that infants who were abused developed an attachment to their abusive parent. The attachment was more likely described as anxious or disorganized, but they were still bonded to the caregiver (Cyr et al., 2010).

The severely alienated child not only expresses rejection of the parent in an absolute manner but also engages in cruel behavior toward the rejected parent, showing little remorse or conscience. Mental health providers should be aware of this research and the notable differences between children who are victims of abuse and those who are victims of alienating behaviors. Clinicians are not responsible for determining the veracity of abuse allegations. They should maintain differential hypotheses until final assessments are completed by child protective agencies, independent evaluators, and/or the court. However, allegations of abuse are a critical aspect of treatment planning, and understanding the characteristics of abuse and alienation will increase the likelihood that the treatment plan addresses the underlying issues causing the child's rejection.

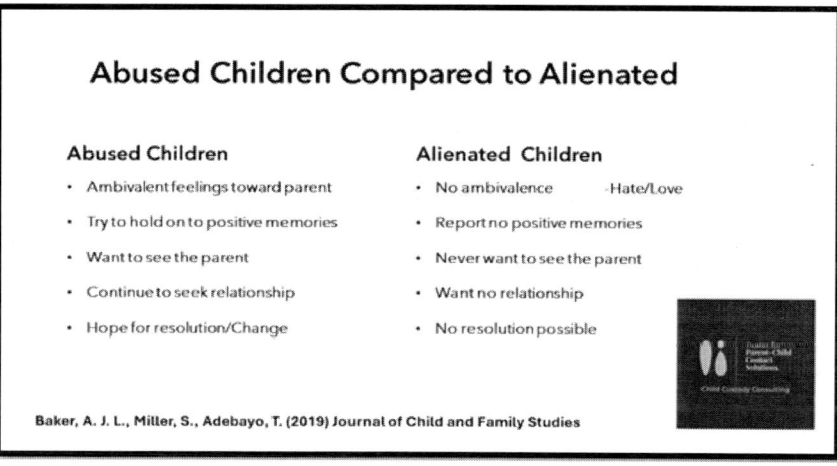

Factor Four

Factor four states that the favored parent has engaged in alienating behaviors. When these behaviors are chronic and long-lasting, they corrupt the child's sense of safety with a caregiver and constitute a form of psychological maltreatment. The DSM-5 (APA, 2013) defines psychological abuse as "Nonaccidental verbal or symbolic acts by a child's parent or caregiver that result or have potential to result in significant psychological harm to the child" (p. 719). The definition includes the following behaviors:

- berating/disparaging/humiliating/threatening/harming/abandoning
- indicating the alleged offender will harm/abandon – people or things the child cares about
- confining the child
- egregious scapegoating of the child
- coercing the child to inflict pain on himself/herself and disciplining the child excessively through physical or nonphysical means

It is not uncommon for parents to behave in ways that are considered alienating during the early stages of divorce. Occasional negative commentary about the divorce or the other parent will not result in parental alienation. If these comments are addressed early on, many parents will quickly understand that their behavior has the potential to do a great deal of damage to their children and immediately discontinue it.

This is diagnostic for clinicians. If a parent receives information about their negative behaviors and the consequences of those behaviors on the child, and the parent can change that behavior, clinical interventions have a much better chance of success. There is increased confidence that the child's resistance will continue to decrease rather than entrench further. When parents cannot receive information about behaviors that are contributing negatively to the child's relationship with the other parent, clinicians can expect that the current level of resistance in the child will continue to worsen. Chapter 7, "Treatment with the Child," offers some suggestions for how to build resiliency in the child when parents cannot or will not acknowledge their alienating behaviors.

Alienating behaviors have been classified into 17 primary strategies (Baker & Fine, 2008). Researchers have found that these strategies can be emotionally manipulative by creating distorted perceptions and negative emotions toward the other parent. These behaviors negatively impact the child's sense of security with the other parent (Baker, 2020). They can also have a negative impact on the child's attachment with the favored parent because the child realizes at some level that the favored parent's love and acceptance is dependent on them disavowing their love for the other parent (Baker & Ben-Ami, 2011). This may partially explain the desperate nature of the alienated child's clinging to and protection of the favored parent, which is more representative of an insecure attachment than a secure attachment (Bowlby, 1988).

Researchers have found that adults who experienced denigration of a parent by the other parent during childhood reported less closeness with both of their parents (Rowen & Emery, 2014), characterized by lower levels of trust, poor communication, more distant relationships (Rowen & Emery, 2018).

The 17 strategies of alienating behaviors are:

1. Bad-mouthing – this includes comments made directly to the child about the other parent and comments made to others (grandparents, doctors, teachers, friends) that are overheard by the child. These comments are rarely accompanied by any positive comments.
2. Limiting Contact – this includes not sending the child during court ordered visitation times, picking the child up early from court ordered visitation time, scheduling appointments, activities that interfere in the child's time with the other parent.
3. Limiting Communication – this includes blocking phone calls, not relaying messages that the parent leaves for the child, blocking email communications, not delivering mail sent by the parent.
4. Interfering with Symbolic Communications – symbolic communications include pictures and storytelling about the other parent. Children need to remember their parents when they are with the other parent. Having family pictures representing good memories is important for children whose parents' divorce.
5. Withdrawal of love – negative verbal and nonverbal expressions when the child talks positively about the other parent or expresses a desire to see/talk/spend more time with the other parent.
6. Telling the child that the other parent does not love them – this was expressed as one of the most destructive behaviors for alienated children, especially when combined with efforts to limit time. The children were easily convinced that this was true when they could not hear statements of love from the parent. This can be expressed indirectly. For example, "your mother enjoys spending time with her new step kids more than she does you or she would have been at your game this morning."
7. Forcing the child to choose – these behaviors include things like asking the child to choose between which parent they want to come to a doctor's appointment or school activity or asking the child to call the other parent and tell them they do not want

to come to their home. The child is asked to participate in the rejection in some way.

8. Creating the impression that the parent is dangerous – this message can be sent directly or implied. This is a form of badmouthing with the specific intent to make the child fear that the other parent will not keep them safe. An implied statement might sound something like, "Your dad is just really forgetful. I used to remind him to put your seatbelt on and not let you run out in the street."

9. Confiding in the child—telling the child about the other parent's faults and sharing adult information about the marriage with the child. The child may come to view the other parent as responsible for the failure of the marriage and problems afterward. They may also feel sorry for the favored parent and be protective of them because they view them as being victimized by the other parent.

10. Forcing the child to reject the other parent – the alienating parent finds ways to make the child feel like they must choose which parent to love, spend time with, or pay attention to. Baker and Fine (2008) provide an example of both parents attending the child's soccer game and regardless of whose parenting time it is, the child feels that they must always stand with the alienating parent. Another example from this author's experience was when the father told the child that she must choose which parent she would celebrate her birthday with because she did not need to have two birthday celebrations.

11. Asking the child to spy on the parent—The alienating parent may be very interested in the other parent's spending habits, salary, and social activities. Children may be asked to send pictures of pay stubs and prescription medicine to the favored parent. This kind of information can be used against the parents in court.

12. Asking the child to keep secrets—The alienating parent may not want the other parent to know about activities and information and will ask the child to keep the information a secret from the other parent. This creates stress for the child because they may feel guilty for keeping information from their other parent. The act of withholding information from the parent can also decrease the closeness in the parent-child relationship.

13. Referring to the parent by first name – can minimize the authority and/or role of the parent in the child's mind.

14. Referring to a stepparent as mom or dad and encouraging the child to do the same.
15. Withholding medical and educational information and leaving the parent's name off registration and enrollment information—these behaviors limit the parent's knowledge of the child's important activities and achievements and possibly cause the child to believe that the targeted parent does not care enough about them to be involved in their education or medical needs.
16. Changing the child's name—Some alienating parents will find a new nickname or abbreviated name to call the child when they are with them.
17. Cultivating dependency – alienating parents engage in boundary violations behaviors (giving the child information about the adult, sharing their emotional experience with the child, etc.), which interferes with the child's development of a healthy sense of autonomy. Alienated children can appear over-empowered, grandiose, infantilized, and/or enmeshed. They often do not engage in developmentally appropriate activities with friends and spend most of their time with the favored parent. Alternatively, they may present to professionals as expecting to be treated as an adult because they have been treated like an adult partner, best friend, or companion by the alienating parent. They are hypersensitive to protecting the alienating parent, often presenting an intense responsibility to defend them. (Baker, 2005; Baker & Chambers, 2011; Baker & Darnall, 2006; Baker & Fine, 2008).

Factor Five

Factor five requires that the child exhibit characteristics typical of alienated children. This cluster of behaviors is unique to alienated children (Gardner, 1998; Saini et al., 2016). Researchers have described them using slightly different terms (Kelly & Johnson, 2001), but the descriptions of the children match the original descriptions identified by Gardner. Thus, the list that most professionals refer to when assessing parental alienation and describing the alienated child is the list provided by Gardner (Bernet et al., 2021). Research studies have validated these eight characteristics as representative of an alienated child (A. Baker & Darnall, 2007; A. Baker et al., 2012; K. Baker & Eichler, 2016; Bernet et al., 2018):

1. Campaign of Denigration—This characteristic refers to the child's tendency (with very little prompting) to profess a litany of denigrating comments about the parent, which can sound very rehearsed, almost like a memorized script. This is most likely observed when the child is asked to speak to a professional related to the case, but it can also occur when anyone (teacher, friend, parent of a friend) asks them about the rejected parent.
2. Weak, Frivolous, or Absurd Reasons for Rejection – the tendency for alienated children to offer reasons for rejection that are typical of most parent-child relationships (bedtimes, homework, chores), absurd in nature (he talks while he is eating, she took our leftover pizza without asking, he sleeps with his mouth open), or normal parenting requests (do your homework before getting on your video games).
3. Lack of ambivalence – this characteristic refers to the extreme polarization in the child's perception of his/her parents. One parent is all good, while the other is viewed as all bad. The child denies any positive experiences with the rejected parent and states that all their experiences are completely positive with the other parent. When shown pictures of positive times (trip to Disney World, holidays, etc.), the child often responds by saying they were "faking it" and pretending to be happy. This is one of the primary differences between an abused child and an alienated child. As referenced earlier, children who have been abused do not usually feel hatred toward the abusive parent. They continue to express an interest in the parent and hang on to positive memories about the parent.
4. Absence of Guilt – this characteristic refers to the cruel treatment that alienated children will exhibit toward the alienated parent. These kids can reduce the parent to tears with hateful words and rejecting behaviors with no apparent remorse or conscience.
5. Independent thinker phenomenon – refers to the tendency for these children to deny that anyone else's behaviors or feelings had any impact on the decisions to refuse contact with their parent. Even when confronted with a scenario where the alienating parent was observed to speak negatively about the alienated parent in front of the child, these children will say that hearing the negative comments had no impact on their negative feelings about the other parent.

6. Borrowed Scenarios – alienated children will often repeat negative phrases, negative stories, and express negative opinions about the rejected parent that are not age-appropriate (e.g., an 8-year-old criticizes the parent for spending too much money on toys), or blame the parent for something that occurred at a time when the child was too young to remember it (e.g., she used to leave me in my crib hungry and crying when I was just born), or engages in logical reasoning and forms opinions that are beyond their cognitive capacity (e.g., 7-year old accuses her mother who is dating of trying to find a man to pay all of her bills).
7. Reflexive Support for the Favored Parent – refers to the alienated child's tendency to jump to the protection of the alienating parent. This occurs with the slightest hint of criticism and even when there is no criticism. For example, the therapist comments on the fact that the child got to have a slushie drink before dinner, as a way of saying, "Oh, isn't it great that you got to have a treat today." The child exhibits anxiety and a need to explain why it is ok that they were allowed to have a treat before they had dinner.
8. Extension of Animosity – beloved grandparents, cousins, aunts, uncles, and family friends of the rejected parent report that the child will not answer their phone calls, texts, or emails or respond to any gifts they send. These extended family members are often people the child has spent holidays, vacations, and extensive time with during the summers. The extension of animosity will also extend to professionals who recommend that the child spend time with the rejected parent and to teachers with whom the alienated parent builds a positive relationship.

As a therapist, you most likely will not have all the information available to you that a child custody evaluator or guardian ad litem does to use the Five Factor Model; however, the elements of the model give you information about what characteristics to look out for when you have individual clients and families who are reporting concerns about alienation. Clinicians can contact other professionals on the case and/or previous therapists and collect additional information such as CPS reports, police reports, and medical records.

The type of information or specific people you need to talk to will depend on the nature of the allegations. For example, if the allegation is that mom frequently had enraged outbursts that involved throwing things at the child or across the room, and the police were called multiple times to the home, the clinician can ask for copies of the police reports. If the child was in therapy when the incident occurred, request a release of information to speak to the previous therapist.

When there is a child custody evaluation or other family assessment being conducted parallel to the therapeutic work, it is more efficient to ask for a release to speak to the person conducting the evaluation. The evaluator will have spoken to the other professionals, reviewed child protection reports, and reviewed police reports. These professionals are tasked with evaluating the evidence and can speak to the likelihood that abuse actually occurred. The treatment chapters will provide advice to clinicians as to how to structure therapy when allegations are still being investigated.

Chapter 5

DIAGNOSTIC CONSIDERATIONS

> **Learning Objectives:**
> 1. Understand when to use the diagnostic codes CAPRD and PCRP.
> 2. Understand the differences in types of parental relationship distress.
> 3. Understand the difference between child loyalty binds and parental alienation.
> 4. Understand the difference between estrangement and parental alienation.
> 5. Understand the differences between mild, moderate, and severe levels of contact refusal.

Children and adults can exhibit emotional, behavioral, and somatic symptoms when dealing with major life transitions such as separation and divorce. When clinical attention is focused on the client's emotional regulation, behavioral issues, cognitive impairments, and/or physical symptoms resulting from relational problems within the family, you should consider the diagnostic codes found in the DSM-5 chapter entitled "Other Conditions That May be a Focus of Clinical Attention" (APA, 2013).

In 2013, "Child Affected by Parental Relationship Distress" (CAPRD) was added to the *Diagnostics and Statistical Manual.* The CAPRD definition provided in the DSM-5 was limited to one sentence stating, "This category should be used when the focus of clinical attention is the negative effects of parental relationship discord (e.g. high levels of conflict, distress, or disparagement) on a child in the family, including effects on the child's mental or other medical disorders" (p. 716). Two of the authors of the DSM-5 and Dr. William Bernet offered an expanded definition and in-depth explanation of the diagnosis in a 2016 article published in *The Journal of American Academy of Child & Adolescent Psychiatry*. This chapter will discuss that article and the appropriate use of this new diagnostic code as well as the other codes in this section of the DSM such as Parent Child Relational Problem (PCRP) and Child Psychological Abuse that may apply to families going through separation and divorce.

Child Affected by Parental Relationship Distress (CAPRD)

Parental relationship distress refers to: (1) chronic bad-mouthing and negative comments by one or both parents about each other; (2) high levels of conflict between the parents; (3) intimate partner distress (IPD); and/or intimate partner violence (IPV). IPD refers to parents who are dissatisfied in their relationship, have poor problem-solving skills, have exchanges characterized by conflict, and perceive negative intentions in their partner. IPV refers to physical conflict such as pushing and hitting, psychological manipulation, and sexual coercion. High levels of parental conflict affect parenting interactions with children and overall parental adjustment. Children experiencing high levels of conflict between their parents are more likely to receive poor discipline, higher levels of negativity, less warmth, and mental illnesses (Beach & Whisman, 2012).

When there are chronic, high levels of parental relationship distress during separation and divorce, it may be referred to as a high conflict separation or divorce. These parents have excessive disagreement regarding parenting time schedules, medical and education decisions, extracurricular activities, childcare, household rules, etc. Their interactions can involve abusive language, threats, and actual or alleged physical violence between the parents or between a parent and a child. It is not unusual for child protection agencies and law enforcement to have been involved. These divorces can take many years of repeated court hearings before things are finalized. Even after finalization, the parents may return to court for repeated modifications of their original agreements (Johnston & Rosby, 2009; Lorandos et al., 2013). In many of these families, the children's entire childhood and adolescent experience may be consumed with court hearings, evaluations, interviews by child protective agencies, and conflict and hostility between their parents.

Impaired functioning in children affected by parental conflict may be exhibited behaviorally (acting out, lashing out, explosiveness, aggressiveness, self-harm), cognitively (conflicting beliefs, loyalty binds, adopting false beliefs about a parent (i.e., parental alienation), affectively (anxiety, depression, post-traumatic stress symptoms) and/or physically (stomach aches, headaches).

The diagnosis of CAPRD is appropriate for children whose parents are still married and for children whose parents are divorcing. For example, if a child's parents are married and they have repeatedly observed the parents engaged in shouting and name-calling, the child may begin to experience anxiety about leaving the parent who seems more vulnerable. The child's anxiety is a result of parental conflict and, therefore, warrants a diagnosis of CAPRD. However, a diagnosis of separation anxiety may also be warranted. Clinicians using both the CAPRD diagnosis and separation anxiety provide contextual information about where the anxiety is coming from, which supports the treatment plan and informs treatment planning for other clinicians working with the family.

This same example could apply to a child whose parents had similar levels of conflict but who decided to separate as a result. Clinicians working with children of divorcing parents may observe their clients desperately trying to maintain relationships with both parents. Loyalty conflicts often emerge during separation and divorce from a triangulation dynamic within the family. One or both parents try to align with the child against the other parent. The child feels anxiety in response to loving two people who do not like each other and may also feel anxiety in response to moving between two parents during exchanges who do not like each other.

The child can cope with the anxiety in various ways: (1) by changing their thoughts, feelings, and opinions based on which parent they are spending time with; (2) by trying to compartmentalize their two homes by never speaking about one parent to the other; or (3) by aligning exclusively with one parent and rejecting contact/relationship with the other. When the child takes on the negative attitudes and beliefs of the favored parent as reasons for their rejection of the other parent, the child's rejection is due to parental alienation. A cross-generational coalition is a form of triangulation identified by family systems theorists Salvador Minuchin (1974) and Murray Bowen (1978). One parent aligns with the child to inflict their anger on the other parent by using the child's relationship with that parent to cause conflict, hardship, and suffering.

In the first two coping strategies listed above (changing their feelings based on who they are with and compartmentalization), the child is attempting to maintain a connection with both parents. In the third option (aligning with one parent and rejecting the other), the stress is too difficult to manage, and there is no way to make both parents happy. The child resolves their internal conflict by aligning with one parent and rejecting the other, temporarily relieving themselves of the anxiety resulting from the loyalty bind, but at significant risk of long-term psychological problems resulting from rejecting a once-loved parent.

As stated previously, when the rejection of the parent was incited by behaviors of the parent with whom the child is positively aligned, such as bad-mouthing and degradation, and the child refuses to have contact because they have come to believe that the parent is dangerous, evil, and/or incompetent, the child is experiencing parental alienation. Children exhibiting parental alienation may have a diagnosis of CAPRD as well as other diagnoses, depending on the goals of therapy. Differentiating between the applicable diagnostic codes is addressed in the following section.

Parent-Child Relational Problem (PCRP) and Child Psychological Abuse

Parent-child relational problems can result from many different issues. The parent may have been absent, intermittently available, overly harsh, abusive, addicted to substances, etc. When these issues have affected the quality of the parent-child relationship, the therapist will use the PCRP diagnostic code when their goal is to reestablish a positive relationship between the parent and the child in either individual or family sessions.

When the clinician is working individually with the child to develop better coping mechanisms for managing parental conflict, CAPRD is the appropriate diagnostic code. A family therapist who is working with the child and the parent attempting to address the internal stress the child experiences from parental discord *and* improve the parent-child relationship should use both CAPRD and PCRP diagnostic codes.

When a parent has been found (by a court or independent evaluation) to have engaged in parental alienating behaviors that caused the child's rejection of the other parent, the clinician treating the alienating parent may use the diagnostic code for Child Psychological Abuse (999.5) when the behaviors of the parent were so egregious to have manipulated the child's memories, perceptions, and feelings about the other parent. Alienating behaviors that cause a child to engage in absolute and total rejection of a once-loved parent are psychological maltreatment and considered emotional abuse (Baker & Veraccio, 2015; Baker & Ben Ami, 2011; Lorandos, 2020; Harman et al., 2018; Friedlander & Walters, 2016).

Interpersonal Violence and Distress

When the child's refusal to see the parent is based on actual events such as abuse, neglect, abandonment, or seriously deficient parenting, the child's refusal is called estrangement. The child may have witnessed the parent being abusive to the other parent during the marriage or witnessed chronic yelling, hitting things, and/or throwing objects. Estrangement is a rational response to a fearful situation. CAPRD and PCRP are still appropriate diagnostic codes for the clinician dealing with estrangement, and the determination of which code to use is still based on whether the goal of therapy is to help the child deal with the stress (CAPRD) or to help the child and the parent repair the relationship (PCRP).

When the focus of the work is with the parents, and the conflict has been characterized by IPD and IPV, the appropriate diagnostic codes are those associated with "Spouse or Partner Violence, Neglect, Abuse – Physical, Sexual, and Psychological" located in the DSM-5 (p. 720-721). Children whose parents are in treatment for IPD or IPV will most likely have a diagnostic code of CAPRD because of the stress and trauma resulting from exposure to high levels of conflict. However, the child may have maintained positive relationships with each parent despite being negatively impacted by their conflict, and in this situation, PCRP would not be used because the relationships are still positive. Other diagnostic codes may also apply, having to do with depression, anxiety, and trauma. The benefit of the CAPRD diagnosis over more general diagnostic codes, such as adjustment disorder with anxiety and/or depression, is that it provides information about the context of the problem, which informs treatment planning.

PARENTAL ALIENATION

A specific diagnosis for parental alienation was considered during the development of the DSM-5. The Task Force acknowledged that parental alienation was a unique and important issue, but they did not think it met the criteria of a mental disorder because it was a problem in the child's relationship with one of their parents as opposed to being an internal condition within the child (Bernet et al., 2016). Additionally, to conclude that a child is experiencing parental alienation requires a more robust forensic investigation than what is expected of individual and family therapists in a private practice setting.

It is important for therapists working with contact refusal to engage in some assessment work to gather as much information as possible to differentiate whether the contact refusal is caused by poor parenting, abuse, absence (estrangement—justifiable rejection), alienation (unjustifiable rejection), or the result of a loyalty bind. The forms of assessment that should be considered are discussed in Chapter 3.

Treatment for contact refusal depends on the reasons for the refusal. Clinicians can cause harm when they treat the contact refusal as alienation and the child's resistance is the result of domestic violence. Likewise, interventions with an alienated child differ significantly from those for children affected by domestic violence. Forensic evaluations are often used to differentiate the causes of contact refusal. Clinicians should wait for the evaluations to be completed to finalize their treatment plan (Polak, 2020; Baker et al., 2020). The authors provide treatment suggestions in the treatment chapters for clinicians who are providing therapy while waiting for the completion of forensic and child protection evaluations. The following diagram may be helpful to clinicians when considering diagnostic codes.

> **Differences and Similarities between Alienation and Estrangement**
>
> | Parental Alienation | Parental Estrangement |
> |---|---|
> | • PCRP diagnosis or CAPRD | • PCRP diagnosis or CAPRD |
> | • Refusal to have contact | • Refusal to have contact |
> | • Lacks legitimate justification | • History of abuse/neglect/seriously deficient parenting |
> | • Driven by a false belief | |
> | • Irrational response to a false belief (maladaptive) | • Driven by real life experience |
> | | • Rational response to an unhealthy situation |

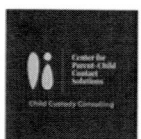

Levels of Resistance and Alienating Behaviors

When working with contact issues, clinicians should assess the level of resistance the child has to the parent and the extent to which the favored parent engages in alienating behaviors, as part of their diagnostic considerations. Resistance is described in terms of mild, moderate, or severe. Documentation of this provides an objective measure of therapeutic progress or lack thereof and should be included as part of treatment considerations.

Mild Symptoms of PA

A child exhibiting mild levels of resistance to a parent may criticize and resist a parent when they are with the favored parent. They may cry or cling to the favored parent at the transition, but once the child makes the transition to the other parent the emotional distress and negativity disappears. The remainder of the parenting time tends to go well, and the parent enjoys normal affection and engagement with the child.

Parents engaging in mild levels of alienating behaviors may be encouraging too much dependency with the child. For example, a mother insists that the father pick the child up from her home instead of from school and, during the exchange, delays the transition by hugging the child repeatedly and lingering. Parents engaging in mild levels of alienating behaviors are usually receptive to education about how their behaviors negatively influence their child. These parents are capable of apologizing to the child, feeling guilt about their behavior, and learning to be careful about what they say in front of the child (Darnall, 2013).

Moderate Symptoms of PA

A child exhibiting moderate levels of resistance to a parent will consistently criticize the targeted parent to people who ask about that relationship (e.g., therapists, evaluators, teachers). The child has a list of reasons why they do not want to or should not have to see the parent. The child's therapist should consider whether these are normal complaints that most kids have about their parents or based on long-standing relational difficulties between the child and parent. Consideration should also be given to whether the reasons are proportionate to their negative emotion about the parent. When the complaints involve abuse allegations, referrals to child protection agencies or law enforcement should be considered (see Chapter 4).

Transitions to the parent the child is resisting may be difficult but do occur. Once at the parent's home, the child may be negative and oppositional. However, they will have some good moments with the parent but refuse to share those positive experiences with the favored parent or their therapist. Therapists working with children in this category will hear about the positive moments from the targeted parent. Regular parent consultations may be necessary to gauge accurately how the time spent with the targeted parent is going (Worenklein, 2013; Gardner, 1998).

Children in this category try to find ways to shorten their time at the parent's home. For instance, they may frequently schedule study groups and sleepovers with friends. They may insist that they need to be at the other parent's home to complete a school project. They may also make frequent requests to begin their time with the other parent a day late.

Parents engaging in behaviors causing moderate resistance are likely to feel some guilt about their negative influence on the child's relationship with the other parent, but they rationalize their behavior or avoid addressing it at all (Darnall, 2013). Some of the most common parental behaviors that cause rejection of a parent are bad-mouthing the parent, expressing anger toward the parent, interfering in the other parent's time, and interfering in the child's ability to freely communicate with the parent, confiding in the child, sharing adult information, scheduling activities that interfere in the child's time with the other parent, and withdrawing love (Baker & Chambers, 2011; Baker & Darnall, 2006).

Severe Symptoms of PA

Children exhibiting severe levels of rejection demonstrate an absolute and total rejection of the parent. In many of these cases, the children have not seen the parent in many months if not years. If the child is still adhering to the court-ordered parenting schedule, they spend most of their time with the rejected parent in their room or away from the home, in school or peer-related activities, and refuse to participate in family activities, meals, etc., with the rejected parent. These kids manifest several of the eight characteristics unique to alienated children: engaging in a campaign of denigration about the parent, acting in cruel ways toward the parent without remorse, giving trivial or frivolous reasons for their rejection of the parent, extending their rejection of the parent to extended family and friends of the parent, stating that their rejection of the parent was their own idea and was not influenced by others, jumping to the protection of the favored parent, lacking normal ambivalence in their relationships with their parents (one good parent and one bad parent), and mimicking negative phrases and messaging of the favored parent when talking about the rejected parent (Warshak, 2013; Gardner 1998). These characteristics are described in detail in Chapter 4. The following diagram conceptualizes the continuum of resistance discussed in this chapter.

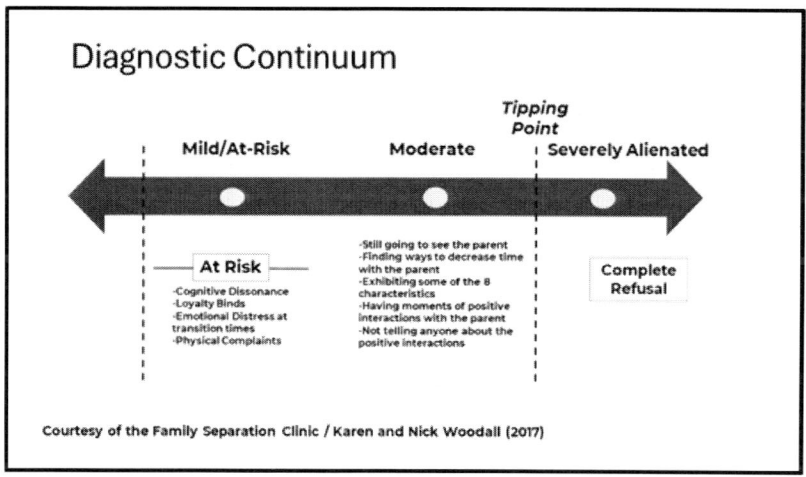

Chapter 6

TREATMENT PLANNING

> **Learning Objectives:**
> 1. Identify the variations in the clinical approach to working with families engaged in active litigation.
> 2. Understand the differential assessment process for treatment planning with this population.
> 3. Understand the special circumstances that surround families in therapy during litigation.
> 4. Understand the limitations in the therapeutic process for families undergoing treatment.

Counseling, psychology, and social work programs attract students interested in making a positive difference in people's lives. The curriculum in these programs is generally based on the premise that the clients we work with want to be there and are seeking assistance to address and hopefully resolve their problems. And yet, this is frequently not the case when working with families involved in divorce litigation.

A fundamental premise of therapy is that psychological healing is grounded in the therapeutic relationship between the practitioner and the client, which is based on unconditional positive regard and trust. To establish this relationship, we are taught processes for building rapport with our clients that include active listening, reflecting, and empathically responding to the information and life narratives our clients bring to us.

While hearing these narratives, therapists are taught to notice incongruent affect, irrational or self-defeating beliefs, and unhealthy behaviors, all of which contribute to the development of the treatment plan. However, we are not generally taught that some clients may purposely distort the facts of their story to gain an advantage in court, deliberately try to sabotage the success of therapy, or consciously hold ulterior motives that run counter to therapeutic goals.

In this chapter, we explore how working with court-involved clients requires variations in the clinician's approach to rapport building. We discuss various resistance behaviors, and describe the differential assessment process required for treatment planning. We conclude the chapter with a discussion about the limitations in therapeutic environments that do not consider the special circumstances of families in divorce and their potential to cause harm to the family.

RAPPORT BUILDING

Assessing Motivation

The authors have found that building rapport with this population should include an assessment of the client's motivation for seeking therapeutic services. Clinicians should consider what the client wants from therapy, how they chose a therapist, and why they thought therapy was something to consider at this time. Is this a parent looking for help for their child? What makes them think the child needs help with issues around divorce? Does the child want to go to counseling? If the therapy is for the parent, what do they want to learn or resolve in therapy? Did their lawyer tell them they needed therapy or that their child needed therapy? Did they call your office because a judge ordered them to? During this initial phase, clinicians should consider the possibility that the client does not truly believe they or their child needs help but is merely doing what they were told. This does not preclude the possibility of positive change, but it does potentially add to the need for specific treatment planning and continued assessment of this issue.

Assessment of the client's motivation includes a level of questioning, even healthy skepticism, that is not typical in the initial counseling sessions with an average client. By questioning, we do not mean literally asking questions about the client's motivation, although that might apply at times; we are referring to maintaining an awareness that the information provided and the behaviors exhibited may be affected by the fact that the client(s) were asked or ordered to work with you, are motivated by an ulterior motive to gain an advantage in court, and otherwise would not seek counseling for themselves or their child on their own accord. This is likely a significant difference in the rapport-building stage than clinicians were taught in graduate school.

Legal Orders

Another significant difference in rapport building is that it should include gathering information about the legal activity occurring simultaneously with the therapeutic work. Treatment is occurring within the context of the legal system. Litigation processes affect the family, and it also affects *and sometimes* directs your work. Your intake information and rapport-building process should include understanding where the family is in the divorce process, who the lawyers are, obtaining releases to speak to lawyers, identifying upcoming hearing dates, and understanding the areas of disagreements between the parents (e.g., What is causing the litigation, who is asking for what, etc.), all of which will help you understand the motivation of your client and dynamics influencing their behavior.

Copies of the most recent court order and/or a copy of the court order outlining therapeutic services should be a part of every client file. The court orders often provide information about how and why the client is seeking services. It may also mandate the frequency of sessions, which the therapist will want to follow. If you have questions about the therapeutic requirements, clarify with both attorneys that your understanding of the orders is accurate. If the attorneys give different answers, correspond with them jointly by email or by conference call and require agreement as to the interpretation of the orders before proceeding.

Clinicians should understand the legal definitions in their state for psychological decision-making and closely examine that portion of the divorce decree or temporary orders when taking on children as clients. In Texas, we have sole decision-making (one parent has the right to decide), joint decision-making (both parents must agree), and independent decision-making (each parent can decide when the child is in their care). If the parents are not divorced yet, they may or may not have temporary orders outlining these rights.

Intake Process

When working with children, it is best practice to include both parents in the intake process, regardless of who has the right to make psychological decisions for the child. The authors never cease to be amazed, even after 25-plus years of providing services, how differently parents conceptualize the issues of the child and the reasons for the child's resistance to a parent. We recommend maintaining as much equal contact with the parents as possible, even when one parent is solely responsible for bringing the child to therapy.

You will come across many situations when this is not possible because a parent does not want to be involved, does not support therapy, does not want to pay for parent consultations, or is particularly hostile and tries to control the therapy. Regardless, both parents should be involved in the child's therapy during the intake process to share information about the child and the relational issues.

Some family members may have fears and personal agendas that decrease their desire for change. They may be willing to follow the court orders for therapy because not doing so would defy the judge and violate a court order. They may be willing to follow their lawyer's advice to get therapy because it would be unwise to go against the advice of their legal counsel, who has likely told them that trying to restore the child's time/relationship with the other parent through counseling is the first thing a court would order. A judge would be highly suspicious that a parent was purposely trying to damage a child's relationship with the other parent if the parent would not agree to therapeutic interventions aimed at restoring the relationship. Resistance to therapeutic interventions can present in several ways, as discussed in the next section. It may be noticeable immediately or become more apparent over time.

FORMS OF RESISTANCE

Licensed mental health professionals are prepared in their graduate training to identify the ways that unconscious resistance presents when touching on deeper emotional issues. This type of resistance is a normal defense when clients process deeper layers of an issue. However, resistance in court-involved clients can be very different. Often, one parent is very motivated to gain the help of a family or individual therapist because they are worried about their child or their relationship with their child. They may have been waiting for an extended period to reach an agreement with the other parent for therapy. They are eager and hopeful that the pain they see in their child and the loss of the child in their own life can be addressed therapeutically. It may also be the case that the other parent, and perhaps the child also, are less eager to start therapy. They may disagree that changes in the child's time with the other parent should be adjusted or that the child should have to spend time with the other parent if they do not want to. In this case, the resistance that interferes with therapy is not the unconscious defense related to deep psychological work. It is a belief or opinion that therapeutic work should not be required, and they are just "checking off the box" to appear compliant.

If the clinician's intake process includes reviewing the court orders, consulting with the attorneys, and conducting parent consultations with both parents, there will be some indicators of each parent's desire for therapy. If the motivation for change is not genuine, tactics for sabotaging success can be detrimental. Many such tactics are obvious, but those used by highly manipulative parents are harder to detect and require clinicians to remain astute to ploys aimed at biasing their view of the other parent or stalling the progress of restoring the parent-child relationship.

Scheduling Issues

Scheduling problems may be the first indicator of resistance to resolution of the parent-child relational issues. Inconsistent appointments, limited availability, frequent cancellations, and intruding on the child's therapy sessions are some of the most obvious ways that parents sabotage therapy. Parents resisting therapy in these ways can cause confusion, chaos, and an immense amount of administrative work for an independent practitioner. Clinicians specializing in this population may want to consider part-time administrative help or sharing the cost of an administrative assistant with another practitioner.

When appointments are canceled, it is common to take 2-3 weeks before another appointment can occur. If this happens a couple of times over six months, the client may only attend one therapy session a month overall. In a situation where a parent is not seeing a child at all or only seeing them in counseling sessions, the loss of parenting time is incredibly painful to the parent, minimally effective (if at all) in creating change in the parent-child relationship, and highly detrimental to the child. Baker et al. (2020) found that a significant barrier to the success of reunification therapy is that practitioners do not hold the favored parent responsible for scheduling delays.

This strategy is of great value to a parent who does not (consciously or unconsciously) want the other parent to have regular custodial time with the child. The agreement to address the parent-child relationship issues in therapy instead of court allows the limited parenting time schedule to continue. For example, if the child has been refusing to transition to the other parent's home, one parent has 100% of the time with the child. If the parent can buy themselves six more months of the same by agreeing to counseling for the child and/or the rejected parent, they are potentially far better off than if they went in front of a judge who might order a regular schedule for the child to spend time with the other parent. In this scenario, the parent's motivation is to maintain the status quo (limited parenting time for the other parent) while preserving their appearance of valuing the child's relationship with the other parent. Therapy is a means to that end, not a quest for resolution and healing.

In this situation, the parent's resistance to the child spending time with the other parent is a root cause of the parent-child contact problem. The court may have to order the parent to have individual therapy, parent education, coparent education, or to participate in family counseling. Their behaviors (resistance) must become part of the treatment plan or be addressed by the court for any change to occur. Still, it could take months of cancellations and rescheduling before their behavioral patterns of interference are clear to the therapist. Keeping detailed records of cancellations and limited availability is imperative, as they will support a request for further therapeutic or educational support for the resistant parent.

Assessing genuine motivation begins with the very first phone call. Parents who have agreed to the child attending therapy but do not, on some level, really want change to occur may use the excuse that their kids are just too busy with school and extracurricular activities to be able to make regular appointments. An initial conversation with this parent may include an extensive list of activities the therapist is expected to adjust their schedule around. When extracurricular activities are prioritized over therapy, therapists must consider several variables to determine whether they are being used as a delay tactic.

Extracurricular Activities

As kids age, they specialize in sports, hobbies, musical, and theatrical activities. Middle school and high school students have after-school activities that are required as part of their course grade. Red flags should arise if new activities are added to the child's schedule at the same time therapy is agreed on or after therapy appointments are made. It is also important for therapists to consider the value of developmentally appropriate activities for a child caught in the middle of a high-conflict divorce. Requiring the child to forego all extracurricular activity for therapy appointments may not be recommended either. A written request to the parents or a recommendation to the lawyers can be made that the parents agree to not add any new activities to the child's schedule for at least three months or some other segment of time that makes sense.

Early signs of resistance manifest in actions that interfere with the start of therapy, such as returning incomplete paperwork, delays in signing consent forms and other required forms, and objecting to standard policy language. This initial stalling often results in a significant delay in starting therapy. It is obvious how this benefits a parent and/or a child who is not genuinely motivated to improve the relationship.

Stalling the Start of Therapy

The attempt to stall the beginning of therapy can be concealed by a parent who expresses enthusiasm and relief for the child or family to begin therapy sessions. In this situation, a parent may leave a message and sound very excited to get sessions set up quickly but then proceed to play phone tag with you for several weeks – forgetting to leave a contact phone number, calling outside of office hours, not leaving a specific time when a return call can be received, etc. This can go on for weeks, and it is easy to lose track of many phone calls that have been attempted. Scheduling notes are a helpful way to track this kind of resistance. Noting these early problems will inform your treatment planning and scheduling processes, which will help keep the therapeutic work as consistent as possible for the family. If, at some point, you are asked why it took so long to start therapy, you will be relieved to have the documentation that confirms your efforts and protects you against claims that you did not follow through adequately.

Parents who are compliant with scheduling but who unconsciously or consciously do not want the child's relationship and time with the other parent restored can interfere with the success of the therapy by trying to control its content. Intrusive behaviors send a message to the child that the content of their therapy is being monitored or somehow influenced by the parent. This can limit their freedom of expression, especially if they need to share behaviors by one parent influencing them to resist contact with the other parent.

Intrusiveness

Parents who request a copy of session notes after every session interfere with the child's privacy and, therefore, limit the topics and feelings the child may be willing to discuss. These parents may request to come in with the child during their sessions or request to speak to the therapist before or after each session. The tendency for that parent to drive the narrative of the child's resistance to the other parent is immense. Therapists should be wary of parents who are overly solicitous and seem intent on giving them negative information about the other parent. We recommend addressing this with the parent and asking them to schedule parent consult sessions to check in on their child's therapy and provide additional information. Parents can send information about the child in an email the day before the session so that there is no interference in the child's therapeutic time.

Maintaining a balanced and accurate view of each parent will require clinicians to involve both parents regardless of who brings the child to the sessions. It is beneficial for the child to observe the therapist communicating with both parents and understand that both parents are involved with the counselor. Avoiding licensing board complaints will require clinicians to maintain consistent communication with both parents; however, the most important reason for interactions with both parents is to limit bias, which interferes with objectivity and accurate assessment of the root causes of the contact issues.

This is one of the most frequent mistakes the authors have seen individual therapists make. When one parent is the only parent bringing the child to therapy, clinicians tend to expect the other parent to reach out to them on their own if they want to be involved or have important information to contribute. However, a parent who has been marginalized does not always think to advocate for themselves, may not consider their perspective important enough to share, or fear that the other parent has denigrated them to the therapist.

Some forms of resistance may only be apparent once the therapist requests that the favored parent make some changes. In this situation, the parent may make all their appointments and speak frequently about how much they want the child's relationship with the other parent to be normalized and repaired. However, when asked to facilitate the child's relationship with the other parent by making behavioral changes, the parent will not be able to do so. Consider the following example:

Case Vignette: Maryann, Rich, Brett, and Brandon

> Maryann brought her two sons, Brett and Brandon, for weekly individual therapy appointments. Rich expressed his frustrations with the prolonged and emotional exchanges between his two sons and Maryann, which occurred every week. The court order outlined that Rich should pick up the boys at the beginning of his parenting time at Maryann's residence. Brett and Brandon were having a very difficult time leaving their mother without a lot of drama, clinginess, and emotional distress. This author recommended that Rich pick the boys up from school instead of mom's residence. At this point, Maryann's cooperativeness and positivity about therapy took an abrupt turn. She was very upset at the thought of not seeing the children before they went with their father, even though this change had the potential of relieving her children from a great deal of stress. Maryann's support for the therapy changed after this recommendation as did her apparent liking of the therapist. Appointments became much more inconsistent.

Karen Woodall (2017), who is an expert in parent-child relational issues during divorce and separation, teaches clinicians that intervention informs assessment. The authors have found this to be true in most cases. You will learn a great deal about resistance as you recommend additional treatment or interventions to restore and increase the child's time with a parent. Often, the very same parents who espouse great support for the child's relationship with the other parent will do things that thwart progress.

Child's Resistance to Therapy

Children affected by irrational rejection (parental alienation) are particularly difficult to work with, as they and their favored parent are not motivated to cooperate with interventions aimed at reuniting them with the rejected parent. Their compliance to therapy is low and they are inclined to act out in a way that sabotages the therapy (Warshak, 2015; Darnall, 2010; Gardner 1998). Their resistance to repairing the relationship with the other parent is clearly articulated to the therapist in the first session. They may provide a detailed list of reasons why they do not want to see the parent, which can range from benign faults in the parent to accusations of abuse, or they may make general statements such as "I just don't feel safe around her," "I just can't relax at his house," or "I just don't want to go over there." Their resistance is rigid and entrenched, and they will have little, if anything, positive to say about the parent. (See Chapter 4 for a full description of the eight characteristics in children affected by parental alienation and Chapter 7 for therapeutic interventions.)

When these characteristics are noticeable, therapists should note them in the record and provide examples of how they manifest in the session. Treatment planning will include decreasing black-and-white thinking, differentiating from the favored parent, and confronting cognitive distortions because these clients are known to exhibit extremely polarized views of their parents. Their negative opinions about the parent have been influenced by the favored parent and are based on exaggerated, false, or incomplete information. Clinicians working with these clients will need to find a way to acknowledge the client's emotional experience without necessarily encouraging the narrative about the parent. Acceptance of the client's narrative, as stated, can lead to inaccurate treatment plans, as the therapist attempts to change something or someone that is not the true cause of the parent-child relational problem. Repeating a false narrative can lead to creating a false memory and continued distortion of the narrative which expands every time the client retells the story (Ceci & Bruck, 1995).

WHY TRADITIONAL THERAPY MAY NOT WORK

A seminal article written by Richard Warshak (2015), entitled "The Ten Parental Alienation Fallacies that Compromise Decisions in Court and in Therapy," outlined beliefs commonly held by mental health and legal professionals working with parental alienation that are not based on the empirical literature and interfere in proper assessment and treatment of the problem. Two that pertain to therapists working in this area and treatment planning are: (1) "Children who irrationally reject a parent but thrive in other respects need no intervention, and (2) Severely alienated children are best treated with traditional therapy techniques while living primarily with their favored parent."

Academic success, commitment to extracurricular activities, and compliant behavior can coexist with serious interpersonal deficiencies and psychological distress that may negatively impact a child's long-term development. Such is the case for a child who is irrationally rejecting a relationship with a loving and safe parent. Irrational rejection is often the result of an enmeshed relationship between the child and the favored parent. The child can feel responsible for taking care of the favored parent, assuaging their anxiety, fears, and sadness, and/or defending them against a parent who they believe treated them unjustly. An adolescent who is enmeshed with a parent may not meet normal milestones that their peers are reaching, such as getting a driver's license, getting a job, and having dating relationships. In all these cases, academic achievements and accolades in extracurricular activities may be present. The therapist should assess peer relationships and other normal developmental achievements as part of treatment planning, even when the client is doing well in school.

Critical thinking skills, conflict resolution skills, and a lack of flexible thinking are typical in children who have aligned with one parent against the other parent. While they may seem extremely capable and compliant in school, they lack the ability to work through relationship conflicts and tend to leave relationships abruptly when conflict arises. This mirrors the way in which they have managed conflict in their parent relationship – severing the relationship to avoid conflict with a parent. Their compliant behavior with teachers and coaches is not generalized to the rejected parent, professionals working with them on repairing their relationship, or with the court. These same children and teenagers exhibit entitled and grandiose behaviors, feeling completely empowered to defy judges' orders and treat the rejected parent in cruel ways without any display of regret or compassion. These behaviors are maladaptive and potentially lead to a series of interpersonal, collegiate, and professional failures as the client enters young adulthood unprepared to function independently.

Traditional therapeutic methods that treat irrational rejection as a phobic response have not demonstrated substantial success (Lampel, 1986; Garber, 2015). Rejection of a parent is often exhibited as anxiety related to being around the parent or anxiety expressed in response to the thought of having to see the parent. Therapists using techniques such as systematic desensitization to expose the child incrementally to the parent may feel confused and disappointed in the lack of progress these children can make as compared to other children who are treated with these techniques for common phobias such as being alone in the dark, sleeping on their own, or spending the night at a friend's home. One reason these techniques are not successful is that many of these children are not actually afraid of their parents.

Mental health professionals who work with children who reject a parent have noted that once the child makes the transition to the rejected parent *and* the favored parent is removed from the environment, the anxiety disappears, and the child engages in normal range behaviors with the parent. In other cases, the lack of anxiety is evident in the aggressive, cruel, and hateful comments made to the rejected parent, none of which are typical of children who are afraid of a parent. Children who are scared attempt to avoid provoking anger in the parent.

Another reason anxiety-reducing techniques may not help these children is that the environment in which they live (i.e., the favored parent's home) does not support or encourage the use of anxiety-reducing techniques with the rejected parent. Favored parents who have encouraged and supported the rejection of the other parent are not inclined to help the child overcome negative feelings that further their agenda of keeping the other parent out of the child's life (Warshak, 2015).

There has been notable research to support that a severe rejection of a safe and loving parent is best treated by time with the rejected parent and time away from the favored parent (Clawar and Rivlin, 2013; Warshak, 2010; Warshak, 2018; Gardner, 2001; Reay, 2015). A therapist has no authority to recommend a custody change or a parenting time schedule change. Therefore, clinicians should realize the limitations in their ability to correct a situation of severe rejection in outpatient settings when the rejected parent has little court-ordered parenting time with the child.

Assessment

One of the differences in treating this population is the more extensive assessment process required before completing a treatment plan (Fidler & Ward, 2016; Fidler, Deutch, & Polak, 2019). Some cases may come to you with a completed assessment, which identifies the causes for the child's resistance toward the parent. However, many families are referred to reunification therapy by a judge or by an agreement between the lawyers, and therefore, the reasons for the child's resistance may not be known. This chapter will focus on the importance of assessment, while Chapter 3 focused on specific assessment activities.

When a family is referred for reunification therapy without a prior assessment, the clinician will need to engage in a process to differentiate estrangement and alienation before knowing exactly how to pursue repairing the parent-child relationship. You can establish general goals based on the intake information presented to you, like improving the child's relationship with the parent, decreasing anxiety, decreasing depressive symptoms, improving peer-related issues, etc. However, your ability to accurately address the root cause(s) for the child's resistance to or rejection of the parent and identify those causes in your treatment plan may require information from other sources. Baker and colleagues (2020) found in a survey of mental health professionals providing reunification services that one-fourth did not conduct an assessment at all, and one-third did not believe it was important to do so.

If there is an assessment occurring simultaneously to therapy, you should approach treatment planning with the understanding that you are waiting on a significant body of information that may impact your understanding of your client(s), your understanding of the family dynamics impacting your client(s), treatment goals, and the techniques you choose to use with your client(s). When there is not an assessment occurring simultaneous to therapy, the therapist should access additional information by asking for information like police reports, child protection investigations, or any other supportive documentation that may exist. Abuse allegations should be taken seriously, and associated information should be explored by the therapist. This may require the therapist to speak to other mental health professionals who have worked with the family and/or review their records. (Refer to Chapter 3 on "Assessment Procedures for Mental Health Professionals (Clinicians)" and Chapter 4 on "Cases Involving Abuse Allegations: Differentiating Between Estrangement and Parental Alienation.")

Identifying and differentiating between the causes for the resistance to a parent will fall to a therapist when there is not an assessment occurring. You may find that a precise understanding of those causes is simply outside the scope of your work, and the best that you can do is outline alternative hypotheses for the possible cause(s) contributing to the rejection/resistance. In this instance, clinicians should not hesitate to recommend a broader assessment to the parents and/or the attorneys, which could explore more fully the causes of the breach in the parent-child relationship.

Working with this population will require clinicians to adjust their intake process to include time for extended assessment activities, such as gathering additional information through documentation and conducting collateral consults. The need for an in-depth assessment is one of the significant differences for clinicians working with this population. It is one of the reasons that traditional therapeutic settings do not often improve the dynamics in these families and why therapists who have not received specialized training are not successful in treating these families and often make things worse (Baker et al., 2020; Warshak, 2015).

Treatment Planning

We have discussed the various ways resistance may be exhibited and stressed the importance of staying attuned to resistance over time. We have also stated that this may require a prolonged approach to assessment. So, how can you move forward with treatment planning when you may have many unknown factors? The chapters dedicated to the treatment of the child, favored parent, targeted parent, and the family provide the reader with specific treatment goals. Therefore, we will discuss treatment goals briefly here from a broader perspective based on some current research of mental health treatment for this population.

Four treatment goals are suggested (Polak, 2020) for clinicians working with parent-child contact issues: (1) Reestablishing contact, (2) improved parent-child relationship, (3) developing a functional parenting plan which includes each parent recognizing how their behaviors contributed to the problems and working to change those behaviors, and (4) developing healthy family functioning which includes managing emotions (usually related to anxiety and anger), improving healthy boundaries, decreasing the child's involvement in the parental conflict, improving healthy communication skills, and improving conflict resolution skills. Baker and associates (2020) recommended resuming parenting time and confronting cognitive distortions as treatment goals.

The three barriers identified as most likely to interfere with treatment success were (1) lack of training in mental health professions, (2) delay tactics by the favored parent, and (3) sabotaging the child's therapeutic relationship with the provider (Baker et al., 2020). Collaboration between mental health providers and legal professionals has been identified as a way to increase the success of treating parent child contact problems (Woodall & Woodall, 2017; Walters & Friedlander, 2016).

Formalized Treatment Agreements

These families appear to benefit from the containment provided by specific formal agreements outlining expectations and goals. Court orders are often written in vague and general language when it comes to therapy. When a court order cannot be written with specific requirements, another formal agreement constructed by the therapist and/or legal professionals can be very helpful.

A structured agreement for the parents should state the overall goals of the therapy, the expectations regarding the frequency of appointments, the parameters of the therapist's role, confidentiality, and fees. While typical paperwork includes statements about fees and confidentiality, the agreement for therapists working with parent-child contact issues provides a different level of commitment and clarification regarding the intent of the work and the requirements of the parents to support the work. These families need containment and structure to deal with their resistance to change. The more structure you can provide at the outset, the less likelihood that sabotaging behaviors by parents and children will interfere in your work.

The agreement also provides a direct and pragmatic way to hold parents accountable. For example, a month into therapy, the child wants to try out for the basketball team at school. The parent with whom the child is most aligned calls the therapist to let her/him know that the appointments may need to be rescheduled because basketball practices will fall on that day each week. The therapist does not need to engage in a protracted conversation about how basketball season could interfere in therapy or try to convince the parent why therapy is more important than basketball. The therapist need only refer to the part of the agreement stating that no new activities will be added to the child's schedule and remind the parent that everyone signed the agreement.

Such an agreement, signed by the favored parent, can also protect a parent struggling to maintain a relationship with the child from being blamed for the child not being able to try out for basketball. Likewise, the therapist's relationship with the child is somewhat protected from the child blaming the therapist or the therapy for interfering in their extracurricular activities. It is not a guaranteed protection from blame, but it does provide some buffer and also provides accountability for the favored parent in terms of setting up a situation (by engaging in any conversation about extracurriculars) that could interfere in the child's relationship with the other parent and/or sabotage therapy.

The authors have found the following agreements helpful in containing the process and guarding against sabotaging behaviors. Many of these were taken from an agreement created by a Canadian attorney specializing in parental alienation, Brian Ludmer:

1. To follow the agreed parenting time schedule (this maintains that the child will continue their schedule even if it is very limited at the time). The agreement should identify the child's current schedule and should be updated if changes are made to the schedule. This helps ensure that the child will not refuse to transition or attempt to decrease their time and that the parent takes responsibility for that (*at least for the time the therapy is occurring*). Therapists cannot enforce parenting time schedules. Including this in the agreement is just an additional imperative to the parent that the current court-ordered time is continuing and the therapy is not used to change it.
2. The parents agree that reunification therapy aims to restore healthy parent-child relationships characterized by healthy age-appropriate boundaries, autonomy, and appropriate parental authority. (This addresses common problems for these families of parentification, enmeshment, overempowerment, and loss of parental authority.)
3. The parents agree that a goal of reunification therapy is to increase their understanding of the negative repercussions of loyalty binds and how their behaviors have created loyalty binds in the children.
4. The parents agree that an overall goal is to increase safe contact between (the parent and the child. *(This does not mean that the therapist will be making parenting time recommendations. It states that*

one of the goals of therapy is to increase the amount of time the child spends with the parent they are rejecting, based on assessments of what is causing the child's rejection.).

5. The parents agree that the therapist will address cognitive distortions and black and white thinking pertaining to one or both parents, leading to more realistic perceptions of the parents.
6. The parents agree that the therapist will help them and their child(ren) to differentiate realistic concerns from exaggerated concerns.
7. The parents agree to learn better problem solving and communication skills to use with each other and with the children.
8. The parents agree to learn how to improve parenting skills and family communication skills.
9. The parents are asked to sign a statement acknowledging that even though they may disagree about what has caused the child's refusal or resistance to see the parent, they are in support of the treatment goals and realize they both play a role in the family's ability to heal and move forward healthfully.
10. The agreement should include a section pertaining to scheduling sessions and should be very specific. This section should include when sessions will begin, how long they will be, how many sessions will occur each week, and what happens if a session is canceled. This may change as the therapist becomes more familiar with the family, so this section should include the therapist's ability to change the sessions and the parents' agreement to adhere to those recommendations.
11. An agreement not to schedule new activities for the child, recognition of the current activity schedule, and an overall commitment to prioritize therapy for at least a certain number of months (3-6 months is standard).

You may find other specific agreements helpful. As you work with these families, your awareness of what tactics undermine your ability to make a positive difference will increase, and you will be able to make changes to your intake procedures and office policies that specifically address those issues.

Chapter 7

TREATMENT WITH THE CHILD

Learning Objectives:
1. Learn the therapeutic foci of treatment.
2. Create therapeutic goals for the child.
3. Learn techniques to use with the child.
4. Learn ways to move forward when progress stalls.

The average child clinician will find themselves in a war zone if working in a high-conflict family without proper training. If you meet with each parent (which you should if possible), the parents cannot agree on much of anything and sometimes even disagree on the symptoms the child is expressing. If the parents are still involved in the court process or expecting to be, you will inadvertently become a weapon that the parents may try to use in their battle and often will become a target.

In high-conflict families, the clinician who refuses to gather a broader perspective about the child's situation will be, at the very least, reinforcing the polarized dynamics of such a family system and, at worst, exacerbating the conflict of the family system and thereby making it a much more toxic environment for their client. Conducting therapy solely on an individual basis with the child tends to be insufficient, as it overlooks the patterns of interaction within the family. Adhering exclusively to this method can inadvertently reinforce the resistance/refusal dynamics rather than effectively addressing the child's best interests.

During the intake process, if a parent is really trying to "sell" their narrative to you, you should see that as a red flag and keep checking yourself to avoid getting too drawn into that parent's narrative. How can you check yourself? If one parent tells you a story that paints the other parent negatively, ask the other parent about their perspective on what happened. If the two perspectives are confusing to you, consider how much more confusing and frustrating it must be for their child to be listening to those conflicting two perspectives on a regular basis. If, for some reason, you cannot speak with the other parent, keep reminding yourself that the other side of the story may be incredibly different.

In any case where you are working with a child of divorce, it is critical that you try to understand the child's complete world they are navigating—what is happening at one parent's house and what is happening at the other parent's house. By limiting your information scope, you may believe you are validating and creating a protected space for your child client. Still, honestly, you are doing a disservice to the child and may only be providing a dysfunctional echo chamber for the child. To be more responsible, you need to be working towards helping the child fit into their own world, and this means that you must understand the realities of the child's world, not simply the child's biased perception of their world (Garber, 2021).

Unfortunately, many clinicians make the mistake of working with children and having very limited information about the child's family dynamic. One could argue that this is unethical practice since ethical guidelines in the counseling fields state one must be competent in the area in which they are practicing (American Counseling Association, 2014; American Psychological Association, 2016), and best practices in working with a child in a high conflict family require that you work with both parents (AFCC, 2011).

Before proceeding with individual sessions with the child, you need to acknowledge that initial sessions will likely concentrate on understanding the beginnings and the evolution of the resistance/refusal dynamic within the family. Both clinical experience and empirical research underscore that a child's refusal to spend time with a parent is a multifaceted, systems-level issue (Johnston, Walters, & Oleson, 2005). In addition to the potential alienating actions of the aligned parent, the child's refusal could also be a consequence of a 'perfect storm' of converging factors (Johnston, 2010). These can include simultaneous estrangement from the rejected parent due to that parent's behaviors, enmeshment with the aligned parent arising from that parent's emotional needs, specific susceptibilities inherent in the child, and other unusual circumstances within the broader family system. Please review Chapter 2, "Causes of Parent-Child Contact Issues," for a more in-depth discussion of the various factors in contact refusal that you should remember as you become more familiar with the family dynamics.

While it may seem easier and more comfortable for the child to cancel one parent out of their lives, in reality, the long-term effects are more harmful than beneficial. Numerous studies have demonstrated that children who have been alienated develop into adults with severe psychosocial disturbances. As children and adults, they have disrupted social-emotional development, social anxiety, and distrust in relationships (Baker, 2005, 2010; Ben-Ami & Baker, 2012; Friedlander & Walters, 2010; Godbout & Parent, 2008). Their attachment is ultimately disrupted with both parents. When they are adults, they are more likely to divorce or break up with a cohabiting significant other and are more likely to become alienated from their own children (Baker & Ben-Ami, 2011).

When you are treating the child who is from a divorced family, your general therapeutic foci include lifting their burden during transitions from home to home, giving them a protected psychological space, and finding their authentic experience.

THERAPEUTIC FOCI OF TREATMENT

Lifting the Burden

Every child experiencing their parents' separation must undergo the challenging task of reconfiguring their relationships with each parent. Instead of relating to their parents as a united entity, they must now navigate distinct and separate relationships with each parent. If they succeed in maintaining close and meaningful connections with both parents, they are likely to adjust more effectively to life after divorce (e.g. Baude et al., 2016). Moreover, the benefits of these robust relationships extend far beyond childhood, offering emotional stability and support throughout the child's life.

However, maintaining these relationships requires the child to bridge the psychological gap between the parents—a concept referred to as "The Transition Bridge" by family therapist Karen Woodall. This metaphorical bridge represents the mental and emotional journey the child must undertake each time they transition from one parent to another. During this process, they must disconnect their attachment from the parent they are leaving before re-establishing it with the parent they are about to spend time with. This is a task they typically must perform regularly, adding to its emotional complexity (Woodall & Woodall, 2017).

The ease with which a child can cross over the 'Transition Bridge' often depends on the parents' relationship with each other. If the parents maintain a low-conflict, supportive attitude towards each other and actively encourage their child's relationship with the other parent, the child will likely find the transition smoother and less distressing.

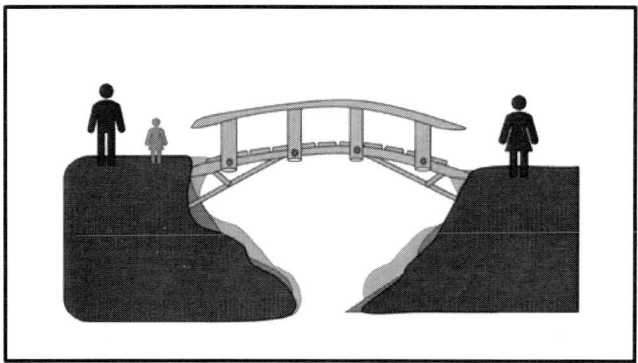

Conversely, if the parents display antagonism towards each other, the child's journey across the 'Transition Bridge' can become significantly more challenging, potentially causing additional emotional strain and complicating the child's adjustment to the new family dynamics (Woodall & Woodall, 2017).

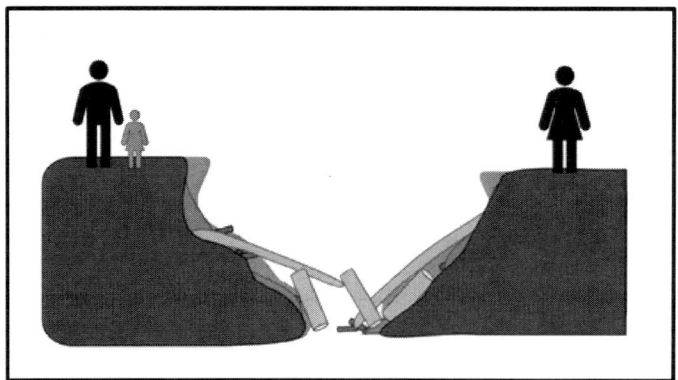

It is important to note that change is hard regardless of whether the change is seen as a positive one. Many parents hang onto the sign that their child does not want to leave their house as evidence that the other parent's house is less desirable. That is not necessarily the case. A child may be very hungry yet reluctant to stop playing a game to eat. Adults may be reluctant to move into a nicer home—not because they do not want to, but because the change process (packing, etc.) is difficult. Just because a child seems reluctant to go to the other house does not mean that they do not enjoy their time once they are there.

Providing Protected Psychological Space

A "protected psychological space" refers to an environment or state in which a child can freely explore their thoughts, emotions, experiences, and relationships without fear of judgment, retaliation, or other negative consequences. In the context of a child undergoing a parental divorce or separation, a protected psychological space is essential to their mental and emotional well-being. This safe space allows the child to process the changes occurring in their family, express their feelings about these changes, and adjust to new family dynamics.

At the onset of therapy, it is important that you operate under the assumption and expectation that a child requires the presence and support of both parents. The ideal scenario is one in which the child is not placed in the position of having to choose between them. Both individual and family therapy aim to create a neutral space where you will promote respect for, and loyalty to, both parents. This balanced approach, which reinforces the importance of both parental figures in the child's life, aims to alleviate loyalty conflicts that the child may be grappling with (Walters & Friedlander, 2010).

A child's relationship with each parent should ideally exist within such a protected psychological space. Regardless of the parents' relationship, each parent-child relationship should be a secure, non-threatening environment insulated from parental conflicts or other external stressors. Some parents can prioritize their child's emotional needs over their feelings toward the other parent. However, many times you may be the only one in a child's life who provides this for the child.

In the therapeutic setting, you can facilitate this protected space by fostering an environment of trust, respect, and confidentiality. The child will be free to love and form attachments to both parents without feeling pressure to choose sides or fear that their relationship with one parent might upset the other. They can express their emotions and thoughts honestly, secure in the knowledge that they won't be used as a weapon in parental disputes or be made to feel guilty for their feelings.

As a clinician, maintaining a firm neutrality stance helps preserve the therapeutic environment as a protected space. This neutrality provides the child with a safe space to explore their emotions away from the pressures of any parental conflict. Your nonjudgmental support can mitigate feelings of loneliness, ambivalence, anxiety, and confusion that can stem from the challenging position of 'being in the middle' (Walters & Friedlander, 2010).

Finding Authentic Experience

Once a protected psychological space is provided to the child, the child is free to go on a journey towards discovering their authentic feelings and experiences. Clinicians are uniquely positioned to offer an alternative adult perspective as their role is distinct from that of a parent. You can interact with the child in a less demanding manner compared to what the child experiences with each parent. When the child is in this protected space free from external pressures and judgment, they can process their emotions more easily (Walters & Friedlander, 2010).

Once a child observes your commitment to the therapeutic alliance and begins to feel secure within this 'protected space, they can often gradually express conflicting emotions and hidden loyalties towards the parent they had previously resisted or rejected. Often children can also acknowledge and articulate mixed or overtly negative feelings towards the favored parent. By reducing their black-and-white thinking, the child opens up to a greater ability for complex thought that is closer to reality. This expanded mental flexibility can have far-reaching benefits, contributing to a more authentic understanding of their feelings and experiences (Walters & Friedlander, 2010).

Mild, Moderate, or Severe

The child resisting or refusing contact with a parent will typically enter your therapy room hesitantly, if not defiantly. As the child's individual clinician, you will need to initially focus on building a strong therapeutic alliance (Smith, 2016). You will also need to assess if the child's resistance to the other parent is in the mild, moderate, or severe range (review Chapter 5, "Diagnostic Considerations"). If the child is in the severe range, it is unlikely that you will make much progress in encouraging him to develop a relationship with the target parent. At that point, you will need to alert whoever is on the legal team of that reality (Warshak, 2020). As an individual clinician, you can pause working on anything directly preparing the child for the reunification process until further support from the court. Instead, you can work on some basic social skills, cognitive distortions, and non-directive work (especially if the child is younger).

There is more hope of positively impacting the target parent-child relationship if the child is in the mild or moderate range. Often, an individual clinician is contraindicated in cases where a child is resisting contact—that is because an individual clinician can make things worse, especially if the clinician is validating the distorted negative narrative the child has of their target parent. You should work collaboratively and in lockstep with the reunification therapist for the best results. If there is not a reunification therapist, it is essential that you do not engage the child much when the child is using you to maintain their negative narrative about the target parent. It is best to stay away from that topic directly and instead focus on general cognitive distortions, critical thinking skills, and emotional regulation unless and until there are some court structures to increase the time between the child and the target parent and/or engage the target parent and child in reunification therapy.

GOALS AND TECHNIQUES OF TREATMENT

When discussing the treatment with the child, the typical goals used for a child in a divorced family and the techniques that can be used to meet these goals will be listed and discussed.

Goal #1—Build Rapport

While this goal may be understood with a child who is dealing with the complexities of their divorced family drama, this is a very important step, especially when you keep in mind how imperative it is for the child to have a protected psychological space.

While it may seem obvious, ensuring a child navigating the complexities of their parents' divorce has a protected psychological space is a critical step in the therapeutic process. The rapport-building process is a key part of creating this protected psychological space. Sometimes, when first meeting the child, you may sense that the child has an agenda, or perhaps it is the parent who brings the child who has an agenda. It's acceptable to allow the child to voice their frustrations or narrative about how they dislike a parent for a while, but it is important that you work on getting that child off that narrative and working on other things. This is part of trying to get them to explore other aspects of their experiences and emotions rather than thinking like one of their parents. This exploration helps the child discover their authentic selves rather than reflecting the attitudes or beliefs of one or both of their parents.

Empathy

One effective approach to facilitating this shift is through empathy. Expressing understanding for the child's difficult situation can create a supportive, validating environment that encourages open communication. Acknowledge their challenges—moving between two homes, adapting to different rules, interacting with different parents, and adjusting to different environments. Your empathy can provide them with a safe space to express their feelings about these transitions and adjustments.

However, if the child completely rejects one parent and refuses any contact (in severe cases), your expression of empathy may need to be more cautious. It's important to validate the child's feelings without reinforcing any negative narratives about the rejected parent. By carefully navigating these conversations, you can help the child maintain their protected psychological space while fostering healthier attitudes towards both parents.

One technique for promoting mutual understanding and empathy in children navigating divorce is showing them videos about other children who have undergone similar experiences. Selecting neutral videos that depict a range of children's experiences during divorce can be particularly effective, especially for children who may be defensive or uncertain about their own circumstances.

One video that has proven helpful, as noted by the authors, is called "What Parents Need to Know from Kids About Divorce," and it is available on YouTube. This video features numerous clips from interviews with children discussing their experiences with their parents' divorce. Another video children seem to enjoy is "The Little Boy and the Beast," available on Vimeo. It depicts two parents who are both initially portrayed as "beasts" who do not like each other and a boy who must go back and forth between them. Towards the end, one of the parents does become less "beastly," and the boy continues to demonstrate patience and compassion toward his other beastly parent.

While viewing either of these videos, the child may wish to comment or share their thoughts. Alternatively, you can initiate a discussion about which parts of the video resonated most with the child's personal experiences. This interaction can provide an opening for the child to share their feelings, understand they are not alone, and gain new perspectives on their situation, all within a non-threatening context.

Building a Covert Therapeutic Alliance

Woodall (2022) discusses the importance of the practitioner building a covert therapeutic alliance with the child. This step can naturally flow once the child feels that the clinician understands them and is most important in cases where a parent is at least partially rejected. As a clinician, you let them know you will take the fall of any positive steps they make with their relationship with the rejected parent, so they do not have to be responsible. In fact, it is often best not to mention these positive strides to the favored parent. Often, a child in this situation will comply with the contact, say positive things about a rejected parent, or even enjoy a therapy session with the other parent, yet then will immediately afterward complain overtly to the favored parent. That is okay. It communicates to you that the child still does not feel like they can be positive about the target parent without consequences from the favored parent. The vignette below illustrates the power of a covert alliance and a protected psychological space.

Case Vignette: Destiny

Destiny, an 8-year-old girl, exhibits significant quietness and withdrawal when transitioning between her parents' homes. Her parents, David and Lisa, frequently argue in front of her, particularly during exchanges and phone calls. This tension affects Destiny, and when she goes to her dad's house, she often withdraws at first and goes into her room before coming out to enjoy her weekend. Her dad reports that she becomes withdrawn again about an hour before going back to her mom's house.

When Destiny first visited the therapy office, she was very quiet and was reluctant to engage in conversation or answer basic questions about herself. The clinician introduced the sand tray to see if she would be interested in playing in that. Destiny seemed to enjoy the sand tray, and soon initiated a game where she hid objects in the sand, prompting the clinician to find them. This game, repeated over several sessions, allowed Destiny to establish control and comfort within the therapeutic setting without direct verbal communication.

Once Destiny seemed more comfortable in the office, the clinician gave Destiny a specific directive: to make an island where she would like to live in the sand tray. Destiny created an island filled with trees, flowers, and various animals, placing herself alone in a chair facing the ocean. At first, she is the only one on the island, as she describes it to the clinician. But then she introduces two figures as her mom and dad, who are swimming in the ocean on different sides of the island. She smiles at the clinician, and the clinician smiles back. From this point on in therapy, she begins to open up about how it makes her feel when her mom and dad fight.

Goal #2—Build Self-Esteem

Self-esteem in a child refers to their internal valuation of themselves, a reflection of how they perceive their own significance and value. Building a child's self-esteem is deeply intertwined with the process of establishing rapport and trust. By encouraging a child to share and teach you about their interests, experiences, and identities, you not only reinforce their self-concept but also convey to them that they are fascinating individuals deserving of attention and acknowledgment. This kind of positive reinforcement instills in them a belief that they have value.

Unfortunately, children who are in a high-conflict divorce where one parent is turning the child against the other parent will be struggling with their self-esteem. Studies show that the more alienation strategies that a child is exposed to, the lower the child's self-esteem. When children are told that a parent is not a good person and does not love or care about them, they appear to conclude that the cause lies within themselves. The favored parent may justify their behavior by saying that they are protecting their child by telling the child "the truth," but in actuality, they are causing harm to the child (Baker & Ben-Ami, 2011).

When a parent exhibits parental alienation strategies, the child's self-esteem is likely to suffer for several reasons (Kruk, 2018). For one thing, bad-mouthing tells the child that the targeted parent does not love them. The child then will believe that they are not lovable. Because of their egocentrism, when they perceive any form of unkindness or lack of affection from a parent, they might internalize the blame, assuming that they are the root cause of such behavior. Feeling unloved by a parent is linked to a decline in a child's self-esteem (Khalique & Rohner, 2002). A child's subsequent self-hatred and depression are linked to both feelings of being unloved by a parent and separation from the parent, and at the same time, they are not able to process the loss of that parent (Warshak, 2015). Hating a parent is unnatural to children and when a clinician sees that in therapy, it is likely due to being taught to the child regularly. If a child has been taught to hate a parent, they will then feel worthless, unwanted, and used in order to meet another person's needs (Baker, 2005, 2010).

A second way in which parental alienation strategies can erode a child's self-worth is through the child's absorption of the negative messages about the targeted parent. Specifically, when they are continually exposed to the notion that one parent is inherently defective or unworthy of respect, the child may deduce that they are also fundamentally flawed as an extension of that parent. In essence, the child believes that if one of their parents is considered "worthless," they must share a part of that worthlessness too (e.g., Greenberg & Mitchell, 1983). Baker's research (2007) with interviewed adults corroborated this perspective. These adults, reflecting on their childhood experiences as alienated children, felt that the "faulty" parent was intrinsically linked to them, both genetically and through the bond they shared. Consequently, they internalized the notion that they must also possess those "faulty" attributes. Thus, the disparagement of the targeted parent by the alienating parent was perceived by the child as a rejection of the part of themselves intertwined with the maligned parent.

Another way by which exposure to parental alienation tactics can negatively impact self-esteem stems from the child's perception of the alienating parent's conditional love. Whether deliberately conveyed or not, the child deciphers that the alienating parent's affection hinges on their acceptance of the negative narratives and subsequent rejection of the targeted parent. Essentially, the child feels that the hatred the alienating parent holds towards the targeted parent outweighs their love for the child. This sentiment often translates in the child's mind as, "I am not worthy of love" (Kruk, 2018).

Techniques

Clinicians have many activities at their disposal to understand a child better and simultaneously weave in therapeutic support and encouragement. One effective method involves using family photographs. By inviting both parents to provide these photographs, the clinician creates an opportunity for the child to explore and discuss their familial memories. As the child shares each photograph with the clinician, they can narrate the stories, emotions, and context behind the images. This offers the clinician a glimpse into the child's past and family dynamics and reinforces the child's sense of identity and belonging. However, it's worth noting that in situations where a child exhibits strong resistance to one parent, this activity might be less beneficial and may even be contraindicated. Conversely, revisiting these familial memories can be a useful therapeutic tool in milder cases where resistance is less pronounced.

Another therapeutic activity involves having the child create an "All About Me" poster board. Begin by providing the child with various magazines, colored papers, markers, crayons, and other artistic materials. Encourage them to sift through the magazines, clipping images, words, or illustrations that resonate with them. They can also integrate their own drawings or doodles, allowing them to express parts of their identity that may not be captured in the magazines. Once the child has arranged and glued their selections onto the posterboard, invite the child to share the significance of each chosen image or drawing. By explaining how each piece reflects an aspect of their personality, interests, dreams, or experiences, the child strengthens their self-awareness and offers the clinician invaluable insights into their inner world.

For more active kids, a ball with questions on it asking the child things about themselves can be helpful. There are countless variations of "All About Me" games and activities, as well as activities created for the specific purpose of building self-esteem, that can be found when buying child therapy tools.

Goal #3—Help Child Individuate from Both Parents

Family boundaries can become unclear in the post-separation environment. These boundaries are needed to establish appropriate roles and authority in the family and create emotional distinctions between family members. In well-adjusted families, there is mutual respect for each member's feelings and needs and clear communication about expectations.

As children grow and mature, their boundaries must evolve to grant them greater autonomy. This allows them to shape their own values, beliefs, and sense of self. In supportive family environments, children are encouraged to gain emotional independence and to develop as distinct individuals rather than an extension of either one of their parents.

In high-conflict divorce situations, the attention to the child's specific needs, including their thoughts, feelings, desires, and requirements related to their developmental phase, frequently becomes overshadowed or diminished (Demby, 2009; Walters & Friedlander, 2010). The risk of enmeshment in these families will thereby increase. This is when boundaries blur, and parents might inappropriately confide in their children or lean on them excessively for emotional comfort. Instead of promoting exploration of their identities, these children might be restrained, not being urged to emotionally grow or distinguish themselves from their parents. Such dynamics can unfairly task children with the emotional labor meant for adults, leading to role ambiguity, placing a parent's needs before their own, and diminishing their sense of identity.

Should signs of enmeshment between the child and a parent become apparent, the clinician seeks to address this complex issue. The clinician's focus is on responding to the child's emotional needs while simultaneously rectifying the child's heightened sensitivity to and sense of obligation for the enmeshed parent, both factors perpetuating the enmeshed relationship.

Techniques

One primary technique will be psychoeducational. The child is presented with the understanding that they are not responsible for the parent's emotional well-being and that the parent does not require the child to need them excessively. These important messages are further reinforced during family therapy sessions with the enmeshed parent (Friedlander & Walters, 2010).

It is essential to assist these children in carving out their distinct identities and separating emotionally from their parents. At the outset, this might be a bit confusing because enmeshment can sometimes resemble a close and healthy parent-child bond. Both the parent and the child might initially struggle. Yet, as therapy continues, the child will deeply benefit as they gain individuality from their parents.

To firmly recenter the focus onto the child, you need to display a sincere interest and a desire to understand the child's unique personality and experience. The child is asked to express their feelings, thoughts, and desires. You, in turn, encourage the child's ability to contemplate how their emotions, thoughts, or desires might differ from those of their parents or siblings. This process promotes the development of the child's individual identity, separate from other family members (Friedlander & Walters, 2010).

In addition to providing psychoeducational support – that is, educating the child about the distinct roles and responsibilities of children and adults within a family system – it is also important for you to explore the child's social skills and relationships with peers. Ideas for questions to seek answers include: Does the child spend time with friends as one might anticipate for someone their age? Do they join in social events or avoid them? Do they have close friendships or struggle with forming lasting connections?

Furthermore, it is essential to investigate the child's involvement in activities suitable for their developmental stage. This involves examining the extracurricular activities the child is involved in. Is the child involved in sports, arts, clubs, or volunteer work that aligns with their interests and age group? Does the child have opportunities to engage independently in activities and events away from their parents?

The process of becoming independent is a critical part of growing up. It involves learning to make decisions, solve problems, and take care of oneself. As such, you should see if the child shows signs of developing independence, such as taking responsibility for tasks, making decisions, or expressing their opinions.

In younger children, this may involve bibliotherapy and some games. Baker and Andre (2015) have a workbook that can help many kids get through the tension of their parents' divorce. The workbook includes an activity focused on the child recognizing and being familiar with their own thoughts and feelings. You do not have to start the activity with their parents as a topic but rather hear their thoughts and feelings on a celebrity, food, popular show, movie, etc.

Another helpful game is to do "Would you rather?" Clinicians can intersperse their questions directly related to the individual case along with more generic "Would you rather" questions. Generic questions could include ones like:

1. Would you rather fly like a bird or swim underwater like a fish without needing to breathe?
2. Would you rather eat only ice cream for a week or only pizza for a month?
3. Would you rather live in a world where animals could talk or where toys came to life?
4. Would you rather have a pet dinosaur or a pet dragon?
5. Would you rather have smelly feet or bad breath?
6. Would you rather spend a day in space with astronauts or at the bottom of the ocean with mermaids?
7. Would you rather always have to hop around like a kangaroo or crawl like a spider?
8. Would you rather live in a giant treehouse in the jungle or a magical castle in the clouds?
9. Would you rather be able to create anything you imagine with LEGO or bring any drawing you make to life?
10. Would you rather play in the world's largest playground for a day or have an amusement park all to yourself for a weekend?

Questions that may be more specific to their situation could include ones like:

1. Would you rather have a week-long vacation with one parent at a time or shorter trips with both parents together?
2. Would you rather spend your holidays alternating between parents or split the day between them?
3. Would you rather have two separate birthday celebrations or one big joint celebration with both parents?
4. Would you rather freely share stories about what you did at the other parent's house or keep each household's experiences separate?
5. Would you rather have both parents attend your school events at separate times or together?
6. Would you rather communicate with the parent you're not with via phone calls or text messages?

7. Would you rather eat your dad's or your mom's best-cooked meal?
8. Would you rather have a fixed schedule with each parent or a more flexible one based on your activities and preferences?
9. Would you rather have each parent keep the rules and routines consistent between homes or enjoy the uniqueness of each home separately?
10. Would you rather celebrate family traditions with each parent separately or create new traditions for each household?

Incorporating music into therapy can be a therapeutic technique when working with an older child or teenager. Encourage the client to explore music that resonates with their emotions. Have them listen to their chosen song while reading the lyrics and engage in meaningful discussions. Some questions to ask might include:

1. How does this song make you feel?
2. Which parts of the song do you find particularly relatable or impactful?
3. Are there any parts of the song that you feel do not align with your emotions or experience?

After discussing one song in this manner, you can further therapeutic exploration by asking the child to select another song that represents the opposite or contrasting emotion. For example, if the initial song expressed feelings of anger, challenge the child to find a song that embodies feelings of peace or tranquility. This exercise can help the client explore and articulate their emotions through music, fostering self-awareness and emotional expression.

Goal #4: Develop Critical Thinking Skills

It is accepted wisdom that when there is outright contact refusal, the child usually holds distorted ideas and beliefs about the parents. Gardner (1998) characterized alienated children as exhibiting an all-or-nothing mentality. Instead of seeing both parents with a blend of strengths and flaws, these children form a distorted reality. In this skewed perception, one parent is idolized as perfect and beyond criticism, while the other is viewed as unequivocally bad.

In a similar vein, Kelly and Johnston (2001) observed that "the child's grossly negative views and feelings are significantly distorted and exaggerated reactions" (p. 254). Similarly, Polak (2019) discovered that most reunification clinicians have reported that children entering reunification therapy often exhibit inflexible thought patterns that may not have a foundation in reality but are shaped by reconstructed memories or perceptions.

Therapeutic support is probable to guide the children towards developing grounded perceptions of both parents. Ensuring their understanding of their parents is firmly rooted in reality is important for their overall well-being (Greenberg et al., 2012).

Techniques

Regarding the particular methods for addressing distortions, Gardner (1998) suggested a direct approach, stating that "At times, challenging the child with illogical and far-fetched claims may assist the PAS child in gaining perspective" (p. 336). Additionally, clinicians are encouraged to express their disbelief regarding the children's negative portrayal of the rejected parent. However, a clinician going too quickly in this manner may find that direct confrontation backfires. If it is backfiring, slow things down. Develop more rapport and try to empathize with the child's perspective. The child's rejection of the parent is often rooted in and justified by these heightened emotions, which block the child's capacity to hold positive thoughts, feelings, or memories about the rejected parent. However, these emotions frequently stem from some level of distortion, sometimes linked to specific events. When you acknowledge, address, and explore these emotions, you are allowing the child to decrease the degree of distortion in their perceptions and replace them with more nuanced and accurate ideas of who their rejected parent is. Part of the therapy process must involve mutual exploration of the underlying causes behind the child's distortions and seeking to understand why the child may have perceived things in a distorted manner before you can start to challenge their belief system (Walters & Friedlander, 2010; Baker et al., 2020).

Most literature focused on therapeutically assisting these children discusses the importance of addressing and rectifying these skewed perceptions (e.g., Lindahl & Hunt, 2016). To foster a healthier perspective, you will need to guide the child from holding stark, distorted perceptions towards adopting a more nuanced and balanced understanding of each parent's strengths and weaknesses (Gardner, 1998; Dattilio & Nichols, 2011; Greenberg et al., 2012; Smith, 2016). Once you've gained their trust, you can then gently start to challenge their thought processes, poking holes in their distortions in a subtle and gradual manner.

Working one-on-one with a child, addressing these distortions in a context outside their immediate family scenario may be more effective. For example, discussing conflicts and intermediation can be approached by examining a scenario where two of the child's friends are in conflict. You could explore how they handle such situations, drawing parallels with their family dynamics, but in a less direct and potentially confrontational manner. This approach allows the child to consider similar issues in a detached context, which can then provide valuable insights and a framework for understanding their own family situation.

Addressing cognitive distortions – or mistaken beliefs – in a child's perception of their family can be a complex and delicate task for a clinician. It's not as straightforward as pointing out the distortions and correcting them; the child likely won't abandon these misconceptions quickly. If you push too hard or fast, the child might cling even tighter to their misguided beliefs, becoming more entrenched in their misconceptions. The more effective approach is to initially empathize with the child, attempting to understand their viewpoint, essentially seeing through their lens.

There are many worksheets and resources specifically designed for children and teenagers that help explore and address cognitive distortions or flawed thinking patterns (e.g., *CBT Toolbox for Children and Adolescents: Over 200 Worksheets & Exercises for Trauma, ADHD, Autism, Anxiety, Depression & Conduct Disorders* (Phifer et al., 2017)). As a clinician, you can utilize these tools to guide discussions with the child. However, when it comes to using examples from their own family dynamics, tread carefully. You should only introduce these personal examples if you perceive that the child is mentally and emotionally prepared to tackle them. Being sensitive to the child's readiness can prevent them from feeling overwhelmed or defensive and promotes a more open and constructive dialogue.

There are strategic moments where it can be beneficial to share certain research findings with the child. For example, discussing how others can influence individual perspectives and behaviors, how personal perceptions can sometimes be skewed, and how our memories might not always be reliable. This approach is rooted in social science research. It can assist in demonstrating to the child that their perception of their family situation, or their views on their parents, might not be entirely accurate. Numerous educational resources like YouTube videos or day-to-day examples can facilitate this understanding (Warshak, 2010).

For younger children, one approach could involve discussing dreams. You might ask if they've ever had a dream so vivid that they questioned later if it was a real experience. You can explain that our minds sometimes struggle to differentiate between what is real and imagined. You could also discuss instances when they might 'remember' a family vacation or an event they don't recall but feel they remember because of frequent family conversations or photographs they've seen. However, it's crucial that these initial conversations are gentle and do not directly tackle any potentially significant distortions in the child's memories or interpretations of their family history (Warshak, 2010).

For older children, more advanced educational content can be used. One powerful resource is a documentary called "Memory Hackers," which details an experiment in which college students were convinced they had committed a crime simply by discussing it repeatedly. This resource could be used to discuss how easily our memories can be influenced and manipulated.

Certain therapeutic books are designed to nurture critical thinking abilities. For example, the book "Tiger-Tiger, Is It True?" (Katie & Wilhelm, 2009) guides children through understanding how thoughts can shape feelings and how, at times, the basis for these thoughts might be unfounded. This concept can be further related to situations where parents might inadvertently or intentionally provide misleading information, leading to negative emotions toward the other parent.

Another game that can be helpful is the Six Thinking Hats (de Bono, 1999), which provides a structured approach to thinking about issues. The method encourages children to approach situations from multiple perspectives, sequentially wearing "hats" of different colors representing a specific type of thinking. Here's how this intervention can be effectively incorporated into therapy to help children develop critical thinking skills:

White hat—What information do we have? What information is missing?

Red hat—How do you feel about this problem?

Black hat—Is it true? Do we know for sure? What could be a problem with this?

Yellow hat—What will happen? What are the benefits?

Green hat—What are some creative ideas for fixing this?

Blue hat—With all of this in mind, what do you think about it?

For example, children can use different hats to express how they feel about a situation (Red Hat), what they think is the root cause (White Hat), the negatives of the situation (Black Hat), the positives that can be drawn (Yellow Hat), and possible solutions (Green Hat).

As you use these techniques, keep in mind that your goal is to have the child decrease their distortions and have a more balanced perspective of their parents and the reality of their situation. In the following vignette, Lily came to the therapy office very aligned with one parent and angry at the other, and her clinician worked with her to be able to have a more complex understanding of both of her parents and was then better able to have a relationship with both.

Case Vignette: Lily

Lily, a 15-year-old girl, has been caught in the middle of her parents' divorce. She comes to therapy initially very angry at her mom, Teresa, for having an affair and destroying their family. Lily's dad, Brandon, has subtly encouraged her viewpoint, enjoying the favoritism he receives from Lily and her younger sister, Leah. He does not share with Lily that he had some infidelities throughout his marriage to her mom. When Lily comes to see her individual clinician to process her feelings, she feels betrayed and is strongly aligned with her father.

As therapy progressed, her clinician introduced the concept that human relationships, including those of her parents, could be complex and how both parents usually have a role in the relationship fallout. At first, the clinician talked about situations Lily may encounter with her peers, requesting that Lily give some examples from her friend situations where one friend may have felt betrayed by another, and they discussed all the dynamics that were going on behind the scenes. Lily started to see how friends can often hurt each other unintentionally or how they may hurt each other because they are hurt themselves.

The clinician then progressed to hypothetical marriage situations where a child may find out that one parent cheated on the other, but, at the same time, some horrible things may have been going on between the two parents without the child's knowledge. Her clinician emphasized that she was not talking about her parents in these illustrations—she was talking about situations that may be similar and may lead a parent down the destructive path of an affair.

Once much of the foundation had been prepared, Lily's clinician decided to have a joint session with Lily and her mom. After apologizing for all the hurt Teresa caused to Lily and her sister by having an affair, Teresa was instructed to be as neutral as possible and open up about her own experiences in the marriage. She shared with Lily how she felt when her dad spent too much time at work or with people at work instead of at home with them. Lily started to remember one of her dad's coworkers with whom he spent a lot of time on the weekends. She asked her mom if she thought her dad had had an affair with that coworker. Her mom admitted she believed so and shared with Lily how she had not wanted to reveal her suspicions to Lily or Leah as she wanted to protect them from further hurt.

This session was a turning point for Lily. She began to understand the complexities of her parents' interactions and the mutual faults that contributed to the marital breakdown. Her clinician helped her explore the impact of holding onto anger and the power of forgiveness and understanding, not as a way to excuse what had happened but as a way to find personal peace. Over time, Lily learned to view her parents as individuals with their own strengths and flaws.

Goal #5–Integrate Psychological Split

Part of the child's therapeutic work in restoring their relationship with the target parent is rediscovering their blocked-off positive feelings for that parent. Splitting is a primitive defense mechanism these children use to make the favored parent "all good" and the target parent "all bad." It illustrates the black-and-white thinking addressed in the previous goal when helping the child address cognitive distortions. As these children often display black/white thinking in how they view their parents (the favored parent is all good while the targeted parent is all bad), It is important to work to integrate the good and the not-so-good about each parent and to develop more realistic perceptions of both parents. In other words, you will be applying what they learned about the cognitive distortions to their own family situation. As they develop the more nuanced views of their parents and more trust in their clinician, the clinician will learn how the child has been protecting their favored parent (Walters & Friedlander, 2010).

Integrating the split often comes after the other work has been somewhat successful when the students' thinking about the rejected parent is not as black and white. On the other hand, you can use some of these activities to evaluate how binary the students' thinking is about their parents prior to engaging in correcting thinking errors.

Techniques

Try to engage the child in discussions about the good things and not-so-good things about each home. See if they can have a somewhat balanced view and develop ideas for each category. One home may be better than the other, but children usually can find something good about each home.

Another topic may stem from their "All About Me" project. How are they like each parent? How are they different? Are they able to see the positive characteristics they get from each parent? It may be good to start new and make a "Me Collage," and as they make that collage, discuss the similarities and differences they have with each parent.

You may also want to talk about their memories of each parent. This can come after you discuss how memories can be changed when you are working on developing critical thinking skills. You can ask them to tell you the positive memories of each parent. See if they can differentiate between what they clearly remember and memories they have heard about or seen pictures from but are not sure if they really remember.

Goal #6–Decrease Anxiety and Trauma Responses

Many kids who are dealing with two parents who do not get along will come into a therapy office with what appears to be a trauma response with a parent. The clinician in those situations mistakenly believes that treatment should be like treatment for a phobia of a parent and recommends systematic desensitization. However, in these cases, this will not work because it is not "trauma with a parent" or even a phobic reaction to a parent; instead, it is a trauma reaction to the conflictual waters they have to navigate as they go from home to home.

Techniques

Children and teens from divorced families need to learn to deal with stressful situations that are unique to their situation. For instance, how can they navigate a performance/sporting event when both parents are there. The clinician must help them develop coping strategies for common and unexpected situations. In common situations, a clinician can work with the child to create a plan and then role-play the plan. Hopefully, there will be a family clinician who can integrate the parents into the plan.

It is also crucial for kids to recognize the signs that they are stressed. Teaching kids to be in tune with their bodies and label their feelings is an essential first step for emotional regulation. The clinician should assess where the kids are in terms of their ability to recognize and label their emotions. If they cannot, activities to help them do so would be a critical primary component of teaching them emotional regulation skills.

Books that can help kids identify emotions and recognize distress:

- *Listening to My Body* by Gabi Garcia (younger).
- *In My Body, I Feel* by Jackie Flynn (younger).
- *A Little Spot of Emotion* by Diane Alber—this collection has many books.
- *Fiona the Flamingo* by Rachel Urrutia Chu and Katie Jeffery.

Games that can help a child recognize emotions:

- Emotions Uno is an adaptation using a regular Uno card deck. Each color represents an emotion, and the color of the last card played by each player tells what emotion you need to talk about—"I feel ___ when…" I use colors that coordinate with the Inside Out characters; sometimes, the kids like to hold an Inside Out character as they talk.
    Red—Anger
    Blue—Sadness
    Yellow—Joy
    Green—Disgust OR Fear

Older kids and teens may enjoy using apps to track their emotions. Apps like Daylio, eMoods, Moodtrack Diary, Moody Me, and Mood Barometer can help them become more self-aware of their mood changes regularly.

Once they recognize that a situation is distressing for them based on bodily cues and thoughts, they will be ready to develop effective coping skills to regulate their emotions. When they have high anxiety levels, they may need to look at grounding techniques. One good therapeutic activity is having the kids create a Coping Bag of different grounding techniques and personalize it to their liking. Ideas of items that could be in this bag include items from the five senses:

- Touch: Chapstick clickable pen, bubble wrap, slime, putty, bath and/or shower bombs, and fidgets in general
- Taste: peppermints, water, tea, gum
- Sight: kaleidoscope, favorite pictures, hourglass
- Smell: essential oils, scented candles
- Sound: playlist, noise-canceling headphones
- Other: coloring books, coloring pencils/markers, bubbles, crochet/knitting supplies

Psychoeducation about how the brain works when in distress can help the kid develop a better action plan to cope in such situations. Explain how emotions are contagious and use their peers as examples. Have them visualize being on the non-moving animal on the Merry-Go-Round while their friends are going up and down around them on the moving animals on the Merry-Go-Round.

If they are far enough along in their journey that they can talk about each parent more realistically, you may want to be more focused on how their parents' emotions are contagious. One activity that can be used is to make a Calming Bottle or a Sensory Bottle where they can initially put glitter in it. To make these, you fill the bottle ¾ of the way with water and then the remaining ¼ with clear glue. You can have them add glitter through a funnel for extra decoration. Then, for the therapeutic part, have them add food coloring – one color representing how they feel and one for each parent. Often, kids will put more food coloring in for the parent with more extreme or contagious emotions. This activity could be used repeatedly as different situations arise, or you can use it once to illustrate to them how their parents can impact how they feel about situations (Allen, 2024). And now they have a calming bottle for their Coping Bag.

Goal #7—Decrease Shame and Guilt

Once children who have been alienated are reunited with their parent, they can feel intense shame and guilt for how they treated that parent. While one parent was manipulating them to hurt the other, they had to suppress any feelings of guilt or shame. Over time, these wounds can profoundly impact their ability to trust others in any relationship (Woodall, 2017). One of the key components in many of the reunification workshops that children attend in cases of severe alienation is a letter to the child from the alienating parent, which helps to relieve the child of the shame and guilt for how they treated the target parent (Harman et al., 2021). While a sincere apology from the favored parent would be the most helpful for the child's healing process, very few favored parents can do this.

As the child's clinician, having a more generic psychoeducational conversation about "Influencers" can be helpful. Engaging the child in a discussion about how they think these Influencers have been successful. Also, engaging them in conversations about how they may feel about certain peers or family members they do not know—how did they decide what they did about that person? Talk about how their parents have influenced their thoughts on more general issues. Educate them about how everyone is influenced to a degree and the most potent influencers in their early years are their parents. If they can understand how they are not at fault for what has happened, perhaps their guilt over what they perceive as their fault can be relieved.

PSYCHOLOGICAL INSTRUMENTS

To assess progress, some clinicians like to utilize some psychological screening instruments to see where the child is in terms of depression (e.g., Children's Depression Inventory), anxiety (e.g., Revised Children's Manifest Anxiety Scale [Reynolds & Richmond, 2008]), self-esteem (e.g., Rosenberg Self-Esteem Scale [Rosenberg, 1965]), or in their relationship with their parents (e.g., Parental Acceptance-Rejection Questionnaire [Rohner, 2005]). If they use these tools in the intake process and then re-assess later as therapy continues, it can measure progress.

Being able to concretely state that the child's depression and anxiety have decreased while their self-esteem has increased throughout therapy can be useful documentation, especially if the case ends up in court. If part of your task is to prepare the child for reunification, the Parental Acceptance-Rejection Questionnaire can be useful. Its structured approach to measuring a child's perceptions of parental behaviors can provide insight into the parent-child relationship dynamics. The PARQ allows clinicians to understand the child's views on their interactions with each parent. The scales of warmth and affection, hostility and aggression, indifference and neglect, and undifferentiated rejection give a broad spectrum of emotional and behavioral assessment.

RECOMMENDATIONS WHEN PROGRESS STALLS

When progress stalls in therapy with a child or teen, it's important to reassess and adapt the therapeutic approach to meet the young client's needs better. Sometimes, if you push too much for the child to do something they are not ready to do, the child will not overtly state their lack of readiness, but you will observe less engagement. In such situations, it is often best to return to where the child is, lean into their perspectives, talk about what they want to discuss, and be less directive. Make sure the child feels heard and understood. Validate their feelings and experiences to enhance their comfort in expressing themselves. Use the child's interests to make sessions more engaging. For example, if a child likes drawing, incorporate art therapy techniques.

Techniques such as mindfulness, breathing exercises, and other stress-relief strategies can help manage anxiety or stress that may be blocking progress. Cognitive-behavioral techniques can also be effective in addressing specific behavioral and thought patterns in older children and teens.

However, suppose you still are having difficulty engaging the child. In that case, the favored parent may be saying things to the child that may be undermining your relationship with the child. Try to determine if that is a possibility. If you think it is, try to have some sessions alone with the favored parent to see if you can get their support in the therapeutic process. Sometimes, if the aligned parent feels heard and validated, they will encourage the child to engage with you, and your sessions with the child will immediately show improvement.

If the child continues to be reluctant to engage in therapy, it may be time to refer to another therapist. Every therapist has a unique style and approach, and not every style suits every child. In such instances, referring to another therapist can be a beneficial next step.

Clinician's Toolbox

- ✗ Videos:
    - "What Parents Need to Know from Kids About Divorce"
        - https://www.youtube.com/watch?v=0TeXNsM9U_g
    - "The Little Boy and the Beast"
        - https://vimeo.com/68851140
    - "Memory Hackers"
        - https://www.youtube.com/watch?v=NfPLTtlo2oY
- ✗ Games:
    - Uno using emotions
    - Would you rather
    - Six Thinking Hats
- ✗ Activities:
    - Going through family photos
    - "All About Me" posterboard
    - Making a Calming Bottle
    - Making a Coping Bag
- ✗ Books:
    - *Getting Through My Parents' Divorce: A Workbook for Children Coping with Divorce, Parental Alienation, and Loyalty Conflicts* by Amy Baker and Katherine Andre
    - *CBT Toolbox for Children and Adolescents: Over 200 Worksheets & Exercises for Trauma, ADHD, Autism, Anxiety, Depression & Conduct Disorders* by Lisa Phifer, Amanda Crowder, Tracy Elsenraat, and Robert Hull
    - *Listening to My Body* by Gabi Garcia (younger)
    - *In My Body, I Feel* by Jackie Flynn (younger)
    - *A Little Spot of Emotion* by Diane Alber—there are many books in this collection
    - *Fiona the Flamingo* by Rachel Urrutia Chu and Katie Jeffery
- ✗ Apps:
    - Daylio
    - eMoods

- Moodtrack Diary
- Moody Me
- Mood Barometer
✂ Assessment Tools:
- Children's Depression Inventory
- Reynolds Children's Manifest Anxiety Scale–2nd Edition
- Parental Acceptance-Rejection Questionnaire
- Rosenberg Self-Esteem Scale

Chapter 8

TREATMENT WITH THE FAVORED PARENT

> **Learning Objectives:**
> 1. Understand the importance of involving the favored parent in the reunification process.
> 2. Learn therapeutic strategies to enable and empower the favored parent to support the child's relationship with the target parent.
> 3. Learn how to manage the obstacles the favored parent may bring to the therapeutic process.

THERAPEUTIC FOCI OF TREATMENT

While the focus of reunification treatment seems like it should be between the targeted parent and the child, the role of the favored parent in this dynamic needs to be addressed when working with the family. Without other therapeutic interventions that engage the favored parent and perhaps other family members, the interventions will not be enough to resolve the parent-child contact issues. In the case of the favored parent, this parent does have a great deal of influence and can wield that influence to improve the relationship between the child and the targeted parent. It is important that the favored parent's therapist is aware of the family dynamics and the child's resistance to the other parent so that they do not worsen the issue by validating the favored parent's behavior that is contributing to the problem (Fidler & Bala, 2020).

Working with the favored parent may be the most challenging part of the process. The favored parent can often present very well and support the process. The adage "actions speak louder than words" must be your mantra when evaluating the favored parent. On the one hand, they may claim to want their child to have a relationship with the other parent, and when they are telling you that they want that, they are very convincing. However, then you notice that they find excuses to keep the child out of appointments with the rejected parent, or they are undermining the therapy in other ways. When you hold them accountable for their actions, you will quickly become the target of their disdain. Remember that these are deeply ingrained patterns of manipulation, enmeshment, and conflict, and they will not disappear without resistance.

The favored parent may initially seem very attuned to their child and will claim that they do not need to discipline their child. This parent claims to know how their child thinks and feels most of the time and may also seem very protective and desire to shield their child from harmful external influences. A therapist who is not savvy about these dynamics may be blind to the skills the favored parent needs to learn, such as boundary-setting and encouraging the child to have a life outside of that parent with other peers and activities (Walters & Friedlander, 2010).

While some favored parents may be able to follow the directives of the clinicians, some may also instigate backsliding in the child (Lindahl & Hunt, 2016). In many cases, the favored parent does not support the reunification of the child with the rejected parent (Albertson-Kelly & Burkhard, 2013), especially in cases of parental alienation where the behaviors of the favored parent have significantly contributed to the child's rejection. If that is the case, you can expect the aligned parent to engage in behaviors that undermine the reunification therapy. The behaviors may include creating difficulties in scheduling the child's appointments with the target parent or even bad-mouthing the clinician to undermine the therapeutic relationship with the child.

Since the success of therapy largely depends on the level of the favored parent's engagement in the process, both parents must be motivated to participate in a program designed to improve their child's well-being and commit to actively engaging in activities that align with therapeutic goals (Templer et al., 2017). Therefore, clinicians will need to find ways to maintain rapport while also confronting unhealthy behaviors.

GOALS AND TECHNIQUES

The favored parent's goals and techniques are largely geared toward supporting the reunification process. Their engagement is important, and their lack of support has the potential to undo any therapeutic progress made.

Goal #1—Follow the Court Order

Favored parents are notorious for not following the court orders on the visitation schedule (Baker, 2008), and usually, they can do so without accountability, which empowers this behavior even more. While this goal often will fall on the legal structure to hold the parent accountable, the therapist can undoubtedly stress the importance of following court orders to the parent. Sometimes a therapist can provide illustrations of other cases that did not go in the favored parent's direction when the favored parent refused to follow the court order. Other times, predetermined court sanctions will be implemented should the favored parent fail to comply (Templer et al., 2017). Even with that information, the aligned parent may still have difficulty following the directives in their court order.

Goal #2—Understand Their Own Family of Origin Dynamics

Patterns of parenting often carry over from one generation to the next. It is common to find disruptions in parent-child relationships when exploring the favored parent's family of origin history. Unhealthy alignments such as parentification, infantilization, or enmeshment may also be evident. In psychoanalytic terms, this is called "transgenerational haunting" and can provide insights into the current family dynamics (Woodall & Woodall, 2017). Engaging the favored parent in discussions about these patterns and how they may have shaped their expectations and behaviors in their own parenting can be a powerful tool in breaking the cycle and fostering healthier relationship dynamics. The following vignette illustrates how Kristen came to realize how her past was negatively impacting how she parented her daughter Christina.

Case Vignette: Kristen

Christina and her dad, Keith, had a strong relationship, particularly through their shared interest in softball. Christina enjoyed spending time with her dad on weekends, and he would often help her out a lot with her pitching game. Kristen, however, had mixed feelings about Christina's commitment to softball and her ex-husband's involvement in their daughter's life.

At 12, Kristen began to express her disapproval of Christina's dedication to softball. She suggested that Christina should focus more on other activities. Kristen also began commenting negatively about Christina's dad, suggesting that he would only spend time with her if she kept playing softball—he would not want to spend time with his daughter otherwise.

By the time Christina turned 13, she had significantly reduced her time with her dad, stating that she had other activities to do with her friends. Her dad had a difficult time saying that she should not spend time with her friends, so he relented. Christina also decided to take a bit of time off from softball.

After a while, Christina and her dad's relationship became strained. Christina barely spent time with him, and Keith missed his daughter. Anytime her dad reached out to her to do something, Christina would get annoyed with him. Keith asked Kristen to agree to let Christina and him have some counseling together to repair their relationship. When Kristen disagreed, Keith found an attorney to file a motion to enforce his time with Christina or get reunification counseling. Since it had been a while since Christina had been with her father, the court ordered her to begin reunification counseling first, which would include the whole family.

While Christina and her dad had their sessions, Kristen began attending therapy to address why she was not comfortable with her daughter having a relationship with her ex-husband. During therapy, Kristen made a significant realization: her father had died in a car accident when she was 13 years old, the same age Christina was when she started to distance herself from her own father.

This revelation was a key moment for Kristen. She began to understand that her distress about Christina having a relationship with her dad, Keith, may have been unconsciously influenced by Kristen's unresolved grief related to her father's sudden death. Kristen's behavior towards Christina and her father mirrored her own unresolved feelings about losing her father at a critical age.

Kristen's therapist worked with her to process her emotions related to her father's death and what she missed by not having a father in her life. Kristen started to realize what Christina would miss without having a father, and she decided she wanted better for her daughter. Kristen started working on how she could encourage Christina's relationship with her dad. Almost immediately after Kristen talked with Christina about what she discovered in therapy, Christina lost all her reservations in her relationship with her dad. Christina resumed having regular time with her father and rediscovered her love for softball, aided by a renewed sense of stability and support from both parents.

Goal #3—Support the Relationship Between the Child and the Targeted Parent

The favored parent will likely have misgivings about the child reuniting with the rejected parent. It is up to you to educate the parent on the benefits for the child to have this relationship and the risks to the child if the child loses it. It is your role to guide the favored parent in understanding the critical importance of the child maintaining a connection with both parents. This involves educating the parent on the significant emotional and psychological benefits for the child in having a healthy relationship with both parents.

A key aspect of this education is emphasizing the concept of attachment, which is fundamental to a child's development. Secure attachment with both parents contributes to the child's sense of security, emotional stability, and overall well-being. You should also address the potential risks if the child is deprived of this connection. These risks include difficulties in forming healthy relationships in the future, emotional distress, and a possible sense of loss or guilt that can persist into adulthood (Baker, 2005; Baker & Eichler, 2016). Understanding the favored parent's family of origin allows you to draw correlations between past childhood experiences and current parenting practices. This process can bring forth unconscious parenting practices that are creating unhealthy alignments with the child.

It may be necessary to point out to the favored parent how they might be unintentionally showing a lack of support for the relationship between the rejected parent and the child. The lack of support may be more subtle (Smith, 2016). For instance, the child may come out of a session with the rejected parent in a good mood and may even share something positive about the session, and the favored parent may then withdraw and be quiet. By doing this, the child is given the message that having a positive experience with the target parent is not a good thing. In this instance, if the favored parent's therapist is made aware of such behaviors, they can coach the parent on how to respond more appropriately to the child's excitement.

Clinicians can help favored parents learn to reinforce the child's relationship with the other parent, such as suggesting the child ask the rejected parent for help on something, sending a picture to the target parent of something the child did, or any other activity that could reintegrate the rejected parent's presence back into the child's life (Smith, 2016). The parent's receptivity to these suggestions may be increased when they feel more positivity toward the other parent.

Clinicians can elicit positive memories from the favored parent by asking what they loved about the parent in the beginning of their relationship. Photos or videos of positive times such as vacations or celebrations that include the target parent and the child can be helpful. The parent's ability to elaborate on how those positive experiences beneficially impacted the child can help shift their emotional state.

Goal #4—Increase Insight and Take Responsibility

Cognitive Distortions

Educating and challenging the favored parent about cognitive distortions may help the parent better support the relationship between the targeted parent and the child. In a study by Polak (2020), over half of the respondents (clinicians) noted that both children and favored parents exhibited rigid and distorted thinking patterns. Increased self-awareness can change the conversations they have with the child about the other parent. Here are some ways that cognitive distortions may present in your office:

Black-and-White Thinking: The favored parent may view their ex in extreme terms, seeing them as an entirely bad parent. For example, the parent might say, "They were always a terrible parent and never did anything to take care of the kids. I always was the one who took them to the doctor's and dentist's appointments," ignoring any times when the other parent was supportive and involved.

Overgeneralization: This occurs when a parent takes a single event or behavior and assumes it represents a consistent pattern. For example, if the other parent was late picking up the child once, a parent might say, "They are always unreliable and never follow through," even if this was an isolated incident.

Catastrophizing: Favored parents often catastrophize about the impact some of the target parent's actions will have on their child. For instance, if the target parent has started dating again, the favored parent may believe it will lead to marriage and destroy their child's life (and may fear the new partner's relationship replacing the one the favored parent has with the child). The catastrophizing parent has difficulty considering less extreme or more likely outcomes.

Mind Reading: A parent might assume they know what the other parent thinks or feels without any evidence. Divorced parents with a lot of conflict may really struggle to give the other parent the benefit of the doubt and often assume the worst. For example, they might believe, "They only want more custody time to spite me," without any concrete proof that this is the case and without any consideration that the other parent may simply want to spend more time with their child.

Labeling: This involves assigning a negative label to the other parent based on their behavior. For example, if the other parent forgets an important date, a parent might label them as "irresponsible" or "careless" rather than considering that it could have been an honest mistake.

Disqualifying the Positive: Even when the other parent does something positive, a parent might dismiss or minimize it. For example, if the other parent has special birthday plans and gives a special gift, the favored parent may tell the child, "He's just trying to bribe you" instead of acknowledging the positive effort. This distortion prevents recognizing any good in the other parent.

Personalization: The favored parent might take the target parent's actions personally, assuming that everything the target parent does is intended to hurt or annoy them. For instance, if the target parent plans a special vacation for the child, the favored parent may think, "They're doing this to make me look bad," when in reality, it could be simply about the child having fun.

Parental Alienation Strategies

Increasing insight into the favored parent involves more than just bringing awareness to the effects of their behavior; it requires a structured approach to helping them recognize and change these behaviors. One effective method is to educate the favored parent about Amy Baker's seventeen alienating strategies, as outlined in her work with Darnall (2006). This psychoeducation process begins by presenting these strategies in a non-confrontational manner to make the person more self-aware.

As you go through each of Baker's strategies (Baker & Darnall, 2006), providing concrete examples of how these behaviors manifest is helpful. For instance, if one of the strategies involves limiting contact between the child and the other parent, you might discuss how subtle actions, such as scheduling activities during the other parent's visitation time, contribute to this. Providing real-life examples helps the favored parent understand the abstract concepts and see how they might unintentionally engage in these behaviors. Sometimes, you may have to address the favored parent directly with the mixed messages the parent gives the child. While the parent may verbally express support for the child maintaining a relationship with the rejected parent, their actions might send a different message to the child—one that tacitly endorses the child's refusal to engage with the other parent (Polak, 2020). Such inconsistencies can create confusion and reinforce the child's resistance to the relationship, so it is crucial that you confront them with the favored parent.

While discussing parental alienation strategies, you may be able to incorporate reports shared by the child carefully. For example, if the child has mentioned that the favored parent often speaks negatively about the other parent, this could be used as a point of discussion without directly revealing that the information came from the child. Instead, it might be framed as a general observation or as something commonly seen in similar cases. This approach helps protect the child from potential backlash while addressing the issue.

It's important to observe the favored parent's reactions during this process. Are they defensive, or do they show signs of understanding their role? This response can indicate their level of insight and willingness to change. If they can admit to certain behaviors, even partially, it's a positive sign that they have a teachable spirit and can make changes. The clinician can then build on this acknowledgment by exploring the underlying motivations for these behaviors and working towards developing healthier parenting behaviors. On the other hand, if the parent does not own their part in the dynamic, you may have to be more explicit with the expectations of the process and document the parent's response, which may include decreased cooperation with the therapeutic process (Greenberg et al., 2016).

The goal is to move the favored parent from a place of defensiveness and justification to one of accountability. If they can recognize that some of their actions have undermined the child's relationship with the other parent, this can be a powerful moment of realization. From here, you can guide the parent in exploring alternative behaviors that support the child's relationship with both parents.

By going through each of these steps, you help the favored parent develop a deeper understanding of the impact of their actions. This ultimately creates a more cooperative co-parenting relationship that benefits the child. This process increases insight and paves the way for meaningful behavioral change.

Suggestibility and False Memories

Another crucial area for increasing insight in the favored parent is through psychoeducation on the concept of suggestibility and its impact on memory formation. Research by Ceci and Bruck (1993) provides a foundational understanding of how children's memories can be easily influenced by how questions are asked or by external cues.

You can begin by explaining the concept of suggestibility in simple terms, emphasizing how young children are more susceptible to external influences when forming memories. The discussion can include examples from Ceci and Bruck's research (1993), demonstrating how leading questions or repeated suggestions can alter a child's recollection of events. For instance, a child might be led to believe that an event happened differently than it did simply because of the way an adult framed the questions.

The therapist can also introduce educational videos that illustrate the phenomenon of suggestibility in action. Videos such as those by Professor Ross (2014) and Shaw (2016) are excellent resources that can visually demonstrate how easily memory can be influenced. Watching these videos together in a session allows for immediate discussion and reflection. The parent can be guided to consider how their own interactions with the child might inadvertently lead to suggestibility. After watching the videos, you can encourage the parent to reflect on their everyday interactions with the child. For example, a simple question like, "Are you okay?" might seem innocent, but it can cause the child to question if something is wrong. By analyzing such interactions, the parent can see how even well-intentioned questions might contribute to the child forming biased or inaccurate memories.

The ultimate goal of psychoeducation is to build greater awareness in the parent about how they communicate with their child and how communication can influence how a child perceives the other parent. Once the parent understands the mechanics of suggestibility, they can be more mindful of their language. You can work with the parent to develop alternative ways of asking open-ended and non-suggestive questions.

Goal #5—Increase Ability to Cooperatively Parallel Parent

The last goal is to enhance communication between the parents. Even if these parents struggle to co-parent effectively, they need to establish a method of communication that minimizes conflict and keeps the child out of parental conflict. A practical approach to begin this process is to ask the favored parent what their ideal co-parenting scenario would look like and then work together to negotiate from that ideal toward a more realistic arrangement.

The favored parent might require education on what constitutes healthy divorce dynamics to understand better their role in creating a positive co-parenting environment. This education can help them recognize the importance of setting aside their animosity towards the target parent and focusing on the child. By learning about effective communication strategies, conflict resolution, and the impact of their actions on the child, the favored parent can begin to see the value in creating a more neutral communication pattern with the target parent. This shift in perspective can help to promote a more supportive environment for the child and more productive communication with the target parent.

The clinician may want to review texts or messages between the favored and targeted parent to understand their communication dynamic. Teaching the favored parent (and target parent) to use Bill Eddy et al.'s (2020) BIFF approach at communication to coparent can be invaluable. BIFF stands for Brief, Informative, Friendly, and Firm. This method is designed to minimize misunderstandings, reduce emotional escalation, and keep the focus on the child. Keeping the communication *brief* helps to avoid unnecessary details that can lead to arguments or misinterpretations. It prevents lengthy, drawn-out exchanges where emotions can easily spiral out of control. By focusing on the essentials, parents can limit the interaction to what's necessary and reduce the likelihood of conflict. Being *informative* and providing factual information ensures that the message is understood and that there is little room for ambiguity. When communication is more *friendly* in tone, it is easier to keep the communication civil and respectful, even in difficult situations. This doesn't mean being overly warm but rather avoiding sarcasm, insults, or any language that could be perceived as hostile. Being *firm* means setting clear boundaries and sticking to them. Co-parents need to assert their decisions without being threatening. A firm stance communicates confidence, reducing the likelihood of continued conflict over the same issues (Eddy et al., 2020).

BIFF communication is designed to be less reactive and more controlled, which helps in managing the emotionality that often exists in co-parenting conflicts. The primary goal of BIFF is to keep the focus on the child. By communicating in a brief, informative, friendly, and firm way, the parents can navigate challenging discussions without getting distracted by previous hurts or relationship conflicts (Eddy et al., 2020). Once the favored parent has learned the BIFF techniques, it may be helpful for the clinician to monitor the parents' communication to ensure that the skills are effectively applied.

A parallel parenting plan involves limited communication where only essential information about the child is communicated. It is a structured approach to co-parenting that allows parents to remain involved in their child's life while minimizing direct interaction with each other (including during transition times). To have a strong one, a clear division of responsibilities and a plan for limited communication are needed. It would also be helpful to pre-plan how specific issues will be handled, such as haircuts, piercings, homework, and child appointments. A parallel parenting plan will allow both parents to play active roles in their child's life while minimizing the chances of conflict.

MENTAL HEALTH ISSUES THAT MAY LIMIT PROGRESS

It can be challenging to work with the favored parent. In mild to moderate cases of parent-child contact issues, the preferred parent may lack emotional resilience when dealing with separation and loss. Many of these parents are dealing with significant mental health challenges that make it difficult for them to regulate their emotions effectively (Demby, 2009; Fidler & Bala, 2010). Mood disorders, such as depression or anxiety, are common among preferred parents, and these conditions can intensify their feelings of insecurity and vulnerability. Anxious parents may project their fears onto the child, leading to overprotection or irrational beliefs about the other parent. Depression can lead to a lack of motivation and energy, which can limit participation in therapy. When these mood disorders go untreated, the parent may become increasingly reliant on the child for emotional support, which places undue pressure on the child.

In cases of severe alienation, the preferred parent usually exhibits traits associated with personality disorders, such as narcissistic or borderline personality disorder. These disorders involve primitive defense mechanisms such as denial and splitting, as well as manipulative and controlling behaviors. The alienating parent views the targeted parent through a distorted lens and communicates these negative perceptions to the child (Bernet et al., 2018). A parent with narcissistic personality disorder may struggle with empathy and likely view the child as an extension of themselves rather than as an individual. A parent with borderline personality disorder may exhibit intense emotions and a fear of abandonment. The child will experience this parent as unpredictable, and the parent will often manipulate the child. These kinds of dynamics can create a toxic environment where the child feels forced to align with the favored parent, fearing emotional repercussions if they show any positive feelings toward the targeted parent.

There is a paucity of research on effective interventions for severely alienating parents as they are resistant to psychotherapeutic interventions and meaningful changes in behavior (Reay, 2015; Polak et al., 2020). Family Bridges is a program to reunify severely alienated children and their rejected parent. The alienating parent is asked to change their behavior as a precondition to having time with their child again. Such a program required by the Court helps to balance the Court's responsibility to secure both the rights of the child and the duty to protect the child from psychological abuse.

Family Bridges developed Aftercare, an educational intervention for alienating parents (Rand, 2023). After 18 years, the Family Bridges Aftercare Protocol is now a "standardized, experiential, educational program designed primarily for the AP and their negative advocates." It is used worldwide in every Family Bridges case (Parnell, in press).

In Parnell's study of 67 children where there was a finding of severe parental alienation (in press), of the children who went through the Family Bridges workshop and whose alienating parents attended the Family Bridges Aftercare, 85.7% of them were able to have access with both parents. On the other hand, if the alienating parents did not attend Aftercare, the children only had a 26.1% chance of having a relationship with both parents. Therefore, it seems that the protocol used in this study could be effective to use with the favored parent in cases of severe alienation.

Overall, the presence of untreated mental health issues and/or personality disorders in the preferred parent creates a challenging family dynamic for clinicians. However, they are likely a significant contributor to parent-child contact issues and, therefore, warrant therapeutic attention. Because the issues are often entrenched and difficult to treat, the clinician working with these parents can be frustrated with a lack of progress. The following section of this chapter provides some suggestions when that occurs.

RECOMMENDATIONS WHEN PROGRESS STALLS

When the favored parent's mental health issues may block their ability to meet the treatment goals, clinicians have some options. It may be beneficial to refer them to a psychiatrist to manage the symptoms medically. When the problems seem trauma-based, referrals for specialized therapy such as EMDR may be helpful. Clinicians needing additional information to determine the nature of mental health issues should request a comprehensive psychological evaluation to inform their treatment approach.

On the other hand, if the favored parent's psychopathology is more severe, and they lack insight into the impact of their behaviors, your task is more complicated. Even if the favored parent is resistant to change, referring them to classes that teach essential skills, such as anger management or dialectical behavior therapy (DBT) skills training, can still be beneficial. These types of instruction can help the parent develop coping strategies, even if they do not fully understand or accept the underlying rationale behind the interventions. At the same time, it is important to protect the child as much as possible, which may require clinicians to report their clinical concerns to the court (or a Guardian ad Litem if one is involved) without making specific recommendations about custody or visitation.

In cases of severe parental alienation, it is not unusual for the favored parent to be unable to make progress. The preferred parent may withdraw from the therapeutic process even if it means losing precious time with their child. Unfortunately, as in the case vignette below of Lorelai, the parent often withdraws from therapy, so it may be up to the child to develop the boundaries and skills to navigate a relationship with a parent with severe psychopathology.

Case Vignette: Lorelai

Olivia's parents, Lori and Kevin, divorced when she was 7. Initially, Olivia was close to both of her parents and enjoyed spending time with each of them. However, as Olivia began to enter puberty, Lori began expressing concerns about her father being a potential sexual predator. Lori communicated her worries to Olivia in a way that made Olivia uncomfortable around her father.

Olivia started to worry that every time her dad looked at her, he was looking at her in a sexual way. As Olivia's discomfort and anxiety increased around her father, she would try to avoid time with her father. Both Olivia and her mom shared her discomfort about her father to her therapist. While her therapist could connect what Lorelai had been telling Olivia to Olivia's feelings, she could not help Olivia consider other interpretations of her dad's innocent behaviors.

As a result of Olivia's disclosures, Child Protective Services (CPS) became involved, leading to an investigation into allegations of sexual abuse. During the investigation, Olivia's visits with her dad were temporarily suspended. The investigation by CPS concluded that there was no evidence of sexual abuse. However, due to the severity of the allegations and Olivia's expressed discomfort, the court ordered reunification therapy to help restore the relationship between Olivia and her dad.

Lori was also involved in the reunification process. She was educated about how she may be putting her anxieties on Olivia. Lori was also coached on how to support Olivia's relationship with her dad. Despite Lori's therapy and the court's orders, Lori struggled to see how her own fears and influence had contributed to the difficulties between Olivia and her dad. She believed she was telling the truth, and only she knew Kevin the way he was. She continued to make negative comments about Olivia's dad, and Olivia even started to refuse to go to joint sessions with him in therapy. Lori's continued alienating behaviors hindered the reunification process, and the reunification therapist had to report the lack of progress to the Guardian ad Litem.

Reunification therapy was stalled due to Lori's refusal to acknowledge her role in the situation. The court decided that Olivia should live with her father full-time and not have contact with her mom until her mom was able to acknowledge her alienating behaviors that hurt Olivia's relationship with her dad. Meanwhile, Lori was ordered to continue therapy to address her issues and the impact of her actions on Olivia before she could begin having normally scheduled time with Olivia again.

Lori maintained that she did nothing wrong. She soon entered into a new relationship and moved out of state. Now, Olivia had to adjust to not having her mom in her life and deal with her new feelings of abandonment. As Olivia continued therapy, she started to have a new understanding of how her mom had influenced her to have discomfort around her dad. Her relationship with her dad grew stronger, and Olivia began to understand how her mom has her own issues and may not be able to ever support her relationship with her dad. When her mom moved back in town two years later, Olivia wanted to see her. She felt like her relationship with her dad was strong enough that she could see her mom without being influenced to fear her dad again.

When faced with a situation where the parent withdraws from the therapeutic process, the primary focus shifts to supporting the child through the emotional difficulties of essentially losing one of their parents. At this point, it would be important to have one treatment focus to help the child build resiliency skills. This involves equipping the child with an understanding of how the favored parent's behavior influenced the child's perception of the target parent. By understanding their favored parent's limitations, they may be better able to set proper boundaries in a relationship with that parent. While this reconnection may be more superficial, they can now interact with their parent in a more balanced way. Ultimately, the goal is to support the child's relationships with both parents, even when the favored parent remains unable or unwilling to change.

Clinician's Toolbox

- ✘ Books:
  - *BIFF for Coparent Communication: Your Guide to Difficult Texts, Emails, and Social Media Posts* by Eddy, Burns, & Chafin.
- ✘ Videos:
  - *Brain Games: False Memory and Misinformation Effect* [Video]. YouTube. https://www.youtube.com/watch?v=qQ-96BLaKYQ.
  - *"Memory Hackers" NOVA* [Video]. YouTube. https://www.youtube.com/watch?v=NfPLTtlo2oY.
- ✘ 17 Alienating Strategies:
  - Strategy 1: Bad-mouthing
  - Strategy 2: Limiting Contact
  - Strategy 3: Interfering with Communication
  - Strategy 4: Interfering with Symbolic Communication
  - Strategy 5: Withdrawal of Love
  - Strategy 6: Telling Child Targeted Parent Does Not Love Him or Her

Strategy 7: Forcing Child to Choose
Strategy 8: Creating the Impression that the Targeted Parent is Dangerous
Strategy 9: Confiding in Child
Strategy 10: Forcing Child to Reject Targeted Parent
Strategy 11: Asking Child to Spy on Targeted Parent
Strategy 12: Asking Child to Keep Secrets from Targeted Parent
Strategy 13: Referring to Targeted Parent by First Name
Strategy 14: Referring to a Stepparent as "Mom" or "Dad" and Encouraging Child to Do the Same
Strategy 15: Withholding Medical, Academic, and Other Important Information from Targeted Parent/ Keeping Targeted Parent's Name off of Medical, Academic, and Other Relevant Documents
Strategy 16: Changing Child's Name to Remove Association with Targeted Parent
Strategy 17: Cultivating Dependency

Chapter 9

TREATMENT WITH THE TARGETED PARENT

> **Learning Objectives:**
> 1. Understand the unique emotional experience of the targeted or rejected parent.
> 2. Learn the therapeutic strategies for resolving ambiguous loss.
> 3. Understand the differences in the therapeutic needs of rejected parents at mild, moderate, and severe levels of alienation.

THERAPEUTIC FOCI OF TREATMENT

Clinical work with the targeted or rejected parent is focused on building trust, providing emotional support, grief and loss, and education. These parents can vary widely in their willingness to trust mental health professionals based on how long they have been without their children and how long they have been embroiled in litigation. Their need for support and motivation will vary depending on these same factors and the kind of support system they have. Many of these parents will already have their own theory about why the child is resisting them. Still, other parents will enter your office in a kind of daze, feeling as if they are living an unimaginable nightmare and not being able to articulate clearly what has happened. The experience of divorce is a loss in and of itself that warrants therapeutic focus. When it is combined with the loss or withdrawal of a child, a specialized approach that recognizes the ambiguity of the parent's experience is needed. Educational topics may include parenting skills, self-care, co-parenting communication, managing interactions with a resistant child, and understanding how resistance may have occurred in the child.

GOALS AND TREATMENT

Goal #1 – Build Rapport and Trust

Acknowledging Their Unique Experience

Building trust and rapport begins with the clinician obtaining a detailed history of how the parent reached the point in their relationship with their child. If the parent arrives at their first session in a state of deep grief or shock, building rapport may begin with holding the space to allow their grief and simple empathic reflections.

You can reflect on how they may feel as if they are living something out of a horrible movie or nightmare. This simple reflection can immediately release much emotion when other people do not understand what they are going through. Few people in the general population recognize that children and teenagers can be manipulated to take sides and reject a parent during divorce. These parents report that family and friends say, "Don't worry, they are just kids; they will come around, leave them alone, and let them figure it out; they will get over it." Alienated parents who are experiencing the loss of a child they have spent years loving and raising are often very lonely in their grief. As this parent's therapist, your recognition of the loneliness, the deep grief, and the utter confusion they feel immediately provides support and understanding that they most likely have not experienced.

Pauline Boss (1999) is a clinician and researcher who studies ambiguous loss, which is described as the physical or psychological loss of someone when others do not acknowledge the loss and no rituals memorialize the loss. Boss' research and therapeutic work with immigrant and divorcing families demonstrated how unresolved loss was intensified by the lack of acknowledgment from other people. She found that an important part of the healing process was allowing the grieving person to tell their story to another who could listen and empathize.

The listener's ability to acknowledge the ambiguity of the loss was also found to be important. The ambiguous losses of a targeted or rejected parent are numerous. Often, the parent does not know when or if they will see their child again, when or if they will get to hug their child again, if the child will ever speak to them again, or if they will ever share in a holiday again. Even when the child is still going to the parent's home, the parent suffers losses around normal affection and everyday family activities like watching movies and eating dinner, creating great sadness for these parents. The initial work with a parent who is being rejected allows the parent to fully tell their story. At the same time, the therapist fully listens and acknowledges their emotional experience and loss of relationship with their child.

These parents can initially present as defensive, guarded, and skeptical, especially when they have worked with several mental health professionals and endured years of litigation. A friend and colleague of the authors describes these parents with the "Four A's" - angry, anxious, agitated, and afraid. Some targeted parents have spent their life savings on litigation and have not seen their child in a year or more. Their anger and fear is a normal reaction to a traumatic experience. They may see you as just another therapist in a long list of mental health professionals whom they have been required to see but have gained no relief from. It would be a mistake to judge them quickly on this initial presentation and assume that their current attitude is the cause for the relationship problems with their child.

Some of these parents have had access to their children restricted because of false allegations of abuse. The court will often restrict access, not because there was evidence proving the allegations were true, but because the other parent claimed it was true. The court thought it was better to exercise caution until an evidentiary hearing could occur. Strong negative emotions from a parent who has been barred from seeing a child for abuse that did not occur should be somewhat expected. Outrage, depression, anxiety, and skepticism can be normal responses to being accused of heinous acts of abuse and having your reputation in the community ruined. As a clinician working with these parents, you can help greatly by acknowledging their anger, affirming their outrage, and giving them a safe space to express it. The experience of being heard may allow them to receive constructive feedback from you so that their emotions are more contained in other places, such as the courtroom or a forensic evaluator's office.

Getting To Know the Child

The parent will appreciate an interest in getting to know the child through their eyes. Initial sessions with these parents can include the parent bringing photo albums or sharing videos and pictures from their phone. This will also give the clinician some insight into the quality of the relationship between the parent and the child, the type of activities they did together, and the amount of time they spent together. For example, if the parent has pictures of all areas of a child's life (educational), extracurricular activities, holidays, day-to-day pictures of childhood play, and vacations) versus only having pictures of vacations, the clinician has some clue that the parent's time with the child was extensive and that they were an integral part of most all the areas of the child's life.

Knowledge of activities the parent and the child did together will also inform the guidance you can give the parent about how to increase or reestablish connection and contact with the child. If the parent taught the child to play baseball and even perhaps coached the child's team, you might be able to come up with some ideas about connecting with the child through baseball. Reconnecting with the child will likely be the parent's highest priority and what they want to focus on in therapy.

Clinicians can help clients with this goal by understanding how the child received love from the parent. Parental love is often conveyed through involvement with the child, shared activities, and learning experiences. Parents can describe what experiences the child seemed to value, thereby identifying what the child may be missing from the absence of this parent in their life.

In severe situations, it is not unusual for the child to reject all past positive memories with the parent and refuse to participate in activities they and the rejected parent did together. The parent's attempts to reconnect through previous common interests will probably not work when this occurs. The parent's sharing of those activities and the positive memories associated with them will, however, provide the therapist with valuable information about the quality of the parent-child relationship, help build trust and rapport with the client, and increase your understanding of the parent.

Showing love and feeling love are two different things, and often, a parent will be able to tell you all of the ways they showed love but not be sure how the child felt loved by them. The authors often use the *Five*

Love Languages book as an example (Chapman 2010). If the parent has not read it, it might be a good homework assignment for them to read the book, identify the child's love language, and process this with the clinician to generate ideas about how to reach out to the child or spend time with them.

Goal #2—Shift from Anger and Betrayal to Empathy and Compassion

Rejected parents can feel hurt and betrayed by their children's behavior. A severely alienated child will treat the rejected parent with disdain and contempt and say horrible things to the parent to try and make them disappear from their lives. They express their hatred without any signs of remorse. This is one of the characteristics of alienated children that make them unique compared to children who have legitimate issues with a parent (Bernet et al., 2018, 2020; Baker et al., 2012; Blagg & Godfrey, 2018; Gardner, 1992).

The parent's reaction to hurt and betrayal should be processed during individual sessions, but we have not found it productive for the parent to express those feelings during the interaction with the child. The authors have seen children/teens reduce a parent to tears with their words during a family session. One such parent was telling their 13-year-old daughter the activities that she most missed doing with her when the child looked straight at her and stated, "Shut the f... up. I couldn't care less about you. I only faked having fun during those things." This type of cruelty without conscience is one of the hallmark features of a severely alienated child. It will shock therapists and bring parents to their knees (Baker & Darnall, 2007).

One way to help a parent in this situation is to explain the bind that the child is in and help the parent see how the child feels as if they have no other option but to try and push them away. Educating the parent about loyalty binds may include some of the information gained from the parent in the trust a rapport building phase. For example, the parent probably shared some ways the favored parent pressured the child to choose one parent over another. Going through these no-win situations from the child's perspective will help the parent shift to an emotional space of compassion and concern. Once the clinician notices this shift, it should be brought to the parent's attention so they become aware of how their internal state has changed toward the child. This is the emotional space they need to work from when interacting with the child.

The concept of the transition bridge was developed by Karen and Nick Woodall (2017). It can be a useful tool to demonstrate to parents how children become so stressed moving between two highly conflictual parents that they eventually refuse to transition to decrease the stress. The bridge and the area underneath represent the psychological space that the child must navigate on their own when going from one parent to the other:

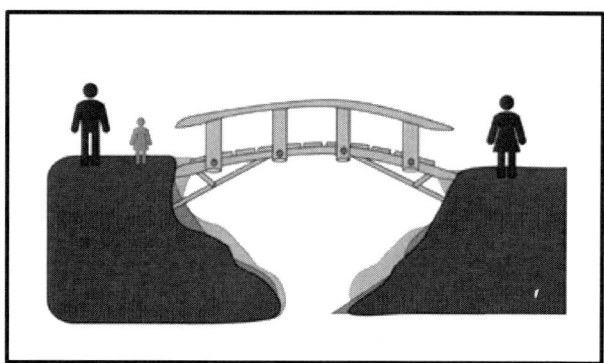

When the child is loaded up with negative feelings and messages about the parent they are going to see, this psychological space can be filled with anxiety, confusion, anger, and doubt as they try to figure out if the negative messaging is true. Using this metaphor, long-term negativity eventually breaks down the child's coping mechanisms and psychological resources. The loss of all ability to cope with the stress is represented by the collapsing of the bridge, which marks the point that the child refuses to transition to the other home.

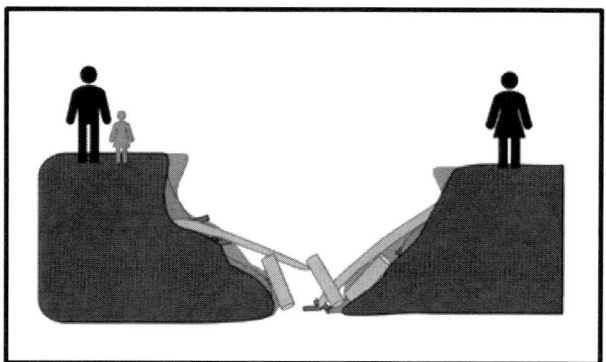

Goal #3—Improve Parenting Skills

Parenting and Parental Conflict

Parenting education can be appropriate when these parents have engaged in overly harsh, rigid, or permissive parenting. In divorce and separation, the element of choice naturally arises for kids. They naturally compare their parents' living environments and parenting. The parent being rejected will likely know what the children's complaints are about their parenting. The therapist working with the parent should help the parent differentiate between frivolous complaints used to bolster the child's case against the parent and complaints with a legitimate basis. The parent's treatment plan should include goals to change problematic parenting behaviors such as overly harsh discipline, non-age-appropriate expectations, emotional nonresponsiveness, and anger, among other parenting characteristics.

Most parents have experienced some form of parenting failure when raising their children. There are no perfect parents, and children often have some real and valid complaints about their parents, particularly teenagers who are beyond their childhood years of idealizing their parents. These parenting flaws do not necessarily warrant the level of rejection expressed by the child but nonetheless can be processed and perhaps normalized in conjoint sessions. Some parents who have struggled with addiction, severe mental health issues, or left the marital home abruptly may have caused emotional pain and need to acknowledge and apologize for that.

The final stages of a marriage can include an escalation of conflict, chronic arguing, and episodes of mild or severe interpersonal violence such as throwing things, slamming doors, pushing, or hitting (Johnston & Campbell, 1993). These situations, even when they are isolated, can be traumatic for the child, and the parent needs to own their part of them when children bring them up as grievances in joint sessions. When alienation is a factor, apologies from the parent may not result in decreased anger in the child, but it is therapeutically important to process the child's experience.

Parenting Alienated Children

Moderately alienated children are often on the cusp of completely severing a relationship with one of their parents. While they may continue to transition between their homes, the parent at risk of losing the relationship with the child will describe their time with the child as mostly unpleasant and may feel as if they are "walking on eggshells" to avoid some conflict that causes the child to completely retreat and refuse to come to their home (Worenklein, 2013). These parents do need strategies for responding to the child's rejecting and often provocative behaviors to avoid a quickly escalating situation that could result in a verbal or physical altercation.

Amy Baker and Paul Fine (2008) authored a paper called "Beyond the high road: Responding to 17 strategies of parental alienation without compromising your morals or harming your child." They provide advice to parents for managing the strategies that favored parents frequently use to disrupt the child's relationship with the other parent. Therapists can use these suggestions to educate these parents on ways to de-escalate conflict and respond to the provocative statements and behaviors of the child. Baker and Fine remind parents to pay attention to the developmental level of the child, to be attuned to the unique characteristics of the child, to be attuned to the alienating parent's unique qualities, to be clear about their own motivations and goals, to have empathy for the child, not to take the bait when the children are trying to provoke an argument, to pick their battles, not to take things personally, and to get support. As we have discussed earlier in this chapter, the rapport-building phase should elicit information about the child that allows the therapist to help the parent identify unique characteristics in the child and the other parent that inform strategies for maintaining a relationship with the child and take into consideration the child's developmental needs.

Developmentally Appropriate Parenting

When the parent has not seen the child in a long while, consider providing education on developmental phases to enhance parenting skills. Developmental changes and cognitive maturity can change what a child needs from a parent. Parents may remember interacting with the child in a way that may not be appropriate now and, if attempted, would only push the child away more. If this is the case, the child's rebuke of the parent's attempts at closeness and connection would not necessarily be because they were alienated or pressured to reject the parent. The clinician working with this parent should help the parent adjust their parenting style to accurately reflect the child's maturity level. A good example of this is the parent who lost contact with their child when the child was 13 years old and does not reconnect with the child until the child is 16 years old. Healthy parenting through these years includes increasing the child's freedom, encouraging more independence, and allowing the child to express their opinions and have input in decision-making. When a parent has missed the gradual steps of increased maturity, they may interpret the teen's resistance as alienation when in some respects it is developmentally appropriate.

Preparing for Reunification

Preparing the parent for interactions with the child is another way to improve their parenting skills. Severely alienated children can act like bullies in therapy sessions with the rejected parent. Reminding the parent that the child will arrive in therapy with the goal of pushing them away is an important part of preparing the parent for the joint sessions with the child. The child is not engaging in therapy by choice. The child is there because someone has told them they must do this, and they would be relieved if the parent decided they did not want to continue the sessions. Therefore, hurting the parent's feelings or behaving rudely and belligerently may sabotage the therapy so that they do not have to attend.

The parent's understanding of psychological splitting as a defense mechanism that protects the child from anxiety and confusion can help them recognize the child's resistance to them as their attempts to protect themselves psychologically from stress. Children engaging in psychological splitting profess to have one parent that they idealize and one that they demonize. If the child acknowledges positive feelings for the "all-bad" parent, they will experience cognitive dissonance and anxiety. At this level of rejection, the child has professed to many people all the reasons they want nothing to do with one of their parents, so to backtrack now could also cause them "face-saving" problems with other professionals, family, and friends. Recommendations for how the clinician can deal with this behavior will be discussed in the treatment chapter on family therapy. The key point here is to prepare the targeted/rejected parent for the behavior and ensure they understand the reasons before interacting with the child.

Goal #4—Increase Feelings of Hope and Empowerment

Once the therapist has determined what level of rejection their client is dealing with, they can choose techniques to help the client stay positive and engaged in activities that give them a sense of control over their world and a feeling of hope that they can make a difference in their relationship with their children. These types of activities usually consist of some combination of (1) ways to increase contact with the child, (2) ways to respond to the rejecting behaviors and maintain connection despite them, (3) building a support system, and (4) self-care and education. The following case vignettes provide examples of a parent dealing with mild rejection behaviors, a parent dealing with moderate to severe rejection behaviors in long-term divorce litigation, and a parent trying to reconnect with young adult children after the divorce litigation.

Case Vignette (Mild): Thomas and Cindy

Thomas had been married for 14 years. He and his wife had a traditional marriage where she stayed home, and he worked. They had one child together. Cindy was nine years old when they separated. Thomas moved out of the marital home and bought a condominium-style home about four blocks from the residence when they decided to divorce. Thomas was an entrepreneur, owned his own company, and had achieved much professional and financial success, allowing him to support Cindy and her mother well and using his time outside of work to enjoy family outings, specialized sporting activities with Cindy, and family trips to many of the national parks in the U.S. Even though Thomas had been busy with work and traveled often during Cindy's childhood, he always thought they had a close and comfortable relationship. Cindy never resisted time with Thomas during the marriage and never expressed anxiety or fear about spending time alone with him. When he moved out of the residence, Cindy came to believe that Thomas left her mom to date other women. In therapy, Cindy revealed that her mother was frequently crying and often told Cindy she was sad that her dad left them and that she believed he might have a girlfriend. Cindy told Thomas that she was uncomfortable spending the night at his home because it was not her real home and because he had not been the parent to raise her because he was always gone for work. Cindy would only agree to spend the day with Thomas every other weekend, and when she came over, she often went through the house and asked why he had things like candles in his bedroom. Thomas was working with Cindy's therapist to try and find ways to help Cindy feel comfortable. He was also seeking his own therapy to help him address his growing anxiety that he was losing his daughter and dealing with the stress of the divorce litigation.

In this example, Thomas' feelings of hope and empowerment could be strengthened by finding ways to stay engaged and involved in Cindy's life, while the divorce process played out. He was having contact with Cindy through her play therapist, who would ask Thomas to participate in her sessions and ask him to bring Cindy to therapy every other week. He also had his parenting time with Cindy every other weekend. Empowering him would consist of finding ways to contact Cindy outside of the weekend visits and being responsive to her questions about items in his household without being defensive.

A clinician working with Thomas will need to identify ways that he and Cindy spent time together when he was living in the home. These activities should be integrated into his parenting time with her. A plan could be created to maintain communication with Cindy between his parenting time. The details of such would depend on the efforts he had already made and what types of communication elicited the best responses from Cindy.

Maintaining involvement in the child's life can involve activities other than direct communication with the child. Even with limited parenting time, parents usually have the right to educational and health information. Parents like Thomas, who have not been responsible for education and healthcare during the marriage, may need encouragement and reminding of their rights to this information. They can schedule parent-teacher conferences, parent consults with the treating mental health provider, and parent consults with medical providers to stay abreast of what is happening in the child's life. These activities are empowering to the parent who feels marginalized and excluded.

Withholding educational and medical information is an alienating behavior. The lack of involvement by the parent in these critical areas of the child's life can create a perception by the child that they have only one parent who really knows or cares about what is happening in their life (Baker & Darnall, 2006). While the responsibility for sharing important information about the child with the other parent generally falls to the parent who has the most time with the child, it is also expected that a parent will take care of themselves to a certain degree and advocate for the information they need to stay abreast of important education and health issues. Parents who stay in touch with teachers, school staff, mental health providers, and medical providers even when they are not having very much contact with the child demonstrate their love for the child, their desire to be involved, and their parenting competence.

The clinician helping parents in situations similar to Thomas's will need to teach the parent how to differentiate between the child's genuine anxiety about spending time with them and irrational rejection generated by negative messaging from the other parent. When dealing with genuine anxiety, making gradual changes to increase time will help the child ease into an expanded schedule. It has been the authors' experience that in the latter situation, when the child is not genuinely anxious but is being pressured to resist parenting time, gradually increasing time only produces more resistance from the child and the favored parent. The parent who can assess this difference knows when being patient is the best thing for the child and when being patient creates more resistance.

Clients in this situation may hear some negative commentary from the kids that appears to have come from the other parent. For instance, Cindy was prone to telling Thomas that she felt safer with her mom because he was gone so much with work. The paper by Baker and Fine (2008) mentioned above offers parents some advice about responding with empathy, hearing the child out, and offering a different perspective to the child. In Thomas' situation, empathy would sound like acknowledgment about how hard it must be for Cindy to get used to spending time with him without her mom, reminding her of all the things they used to do together that did not include her mom and acknowledging that they all have to get used to a new way of being together and assure her that he loves her and will do whatever it takes to help her feel comfortable.

Parents who feel sabotaged by the other parent can become angry about the other parent's behavior (understandably) and miss an opportunity to connect with the child because they are focused on defending themselves against the negative messaging. Defensive and reactive words can increase anxiety in children and increase their resistance to spending time with the parent who comes across as angry and disgruntled instead of calm, grounded, and understanding.

Case Vignette (Moderate to Severe) – Rachel and Justin

Rachel had been married for 20 years. She was professionally successful and had also been the parent in the marriage and was responsible for most of the childcare duties. Her husband worked in sales and made a good salary at times, but he frequently changed employers. His passion was golf, and he hoped to progress from his college golf team to the professional level. This did not happen, but he continued to teach golf at the local country club. Rachel found out that her husband was having an affair and confronted him. She wanted to stay together and asked if they could attend marriage counseling. He agreed to counseling but did not stop the affair. Justin was 15 years old at the time his father's affair was discovered. His younger sister was only 8 years old. Justin's dad began telling him how unhappy he was in the marriage during their weekend golf outings. He shared with him all the things Justin's mom did that made him feel trapped and controlled. Justin began to view his mother's parenting as controlling and began defying her for even minor requests she would make. After about six months of unsuccessful counseling, Rachel asked Justin's dad to move out. Justin blamed Rachel for the divorce and insisted on living with his dad. Once Justin moved to his father's apartment, he refused to return to Rachel's home. Justin eventually refused to accept her phone calls or texts. Rachel believed that Justin had been influenced by his father before the separation. She decided to ask for a custody evaluation in hopes that she could retain primary custody of both children, for fear that if she let Justin go, he would choose not to have a relationship with her. A year and four court hearings later, she was emotionally exhausted. Justin had been moved back to her home by the judge, and his time with his father was restricted while she and Justin had intensive reunification therapy. She had some initial success with Justin once his time with his dad was restricted. They took a summer trip together, and Justin was much like his old self with her. When the school year resumed, Justin began using the school computers to talk to his dad, and his raging episodes with Rachel returned. Rachel was seeking therapy as an adjunct to the reunification work, and she wanted help maintaining her gains over the summer with Justin. She also wanted guidance for navigating her relationship with Justin when the court restored his time with his father.

In this second case example, Rachel went through a year of multiple court hearings and had custody of an extremely angry and defiant older teenage boy. She was tired and running out of energy and money. She needed to find ways to replenish herself and manage the volatility in her son without pushing him away. A therapist helping Rachel work on hope and empowerment would need to hear Rachel's story to understand where she was emotionally and know how to help her. She had multiple layers of loss to process and chronic stress – the betrayal in her marriage, the initial rejection and expressed hatred from her son Justin, the stress of multiple court hearings, the soaring feelings of hope when she reconnected with Justin and gained custody, and then the devastating sense of loss as Justin began to retreat into anger again after having contact with his dad.

Rachel had been in reunification therapy, so she already possessed a good repertoire of responses to Justin's critical and provocative statements. She needed help finding ways to respond to him that preserved her self-esteem, acknowledged his anger, and set appropriate boundaries for him. Staying connected to Justin might include activities they had enjoyed, but it could also be more forward-looking and specific to helping him move into young adulthood.

When teenagers have post-high school goals, activities that help them pursue their options are ways for targeted parents to maintain connection, further healthy development, and stay involved. College trips can be an amazing way for parents to help the teen move into the next phase of their life. Activities such as researching colleges, appointments with financial aid counselors, opening checking accounts, and getting a part-time job are other examples of how parents can stay involved in parenting activities that help the child but have nothing to do with the separation and divorce.

Rachel's therapeutic work should be focused on managing a moderately alienated child (one who is present physically but behaving in rejecting ways) and should also include developmentally appropriate responses for older teens. Rachel's protracted divorce was depleting her. She needed to replenish her emotional reserves to get through the final stages of the divorce and maintain a connection with Justin. Self-care is often an area that parents overlook when they are juggling litigation and resistant teens. These parents are often under the microscope of court-appointed professionals, lawyers, mental health professionals, and the other parent who is looking for any reason to say the kids need to be placed back in their custody. This stress can go on for months as they wait for final hearings or reports from professionals. Clients are unique in how they replenish themselves, and therapists can get creative when helping clients build self-care plans. It is important to give clients permission to focus on their own needs.

Case Vignette (Post Litigation/Adult Children): Amy, Devan, and Maddie

Amy had been married to an emotionally and verbally abusive man for over 20 years. The controlling dynamics in the marriage took a toll on her mental health, and eventually, she ended up hospitalized for a major depressive episode. When this happened, her kids were 17 and 15 years old. Devan and Maddie were encouraged by their father to see Amy's depression as embarrassing and judged her to be an incompetent mother because of it. Their father began lavishing them with gifts, such as travel experiences and cars, after Amy moved out of the family home. Amy decided to separate and divorce after realizing when she was hospitalized that his abusive behavior contributed to her depressive episode. She could not afford to maintain the home, so she was the parent who had to move out and establish a separate residence. Devan and Maddie refused to see her. Devan told her she could not attend his basketball games at the school because he was embarrassed by her. Maddie quit accepting her calls and said she did not feel safe with her for fear that she would have another mental breakdown. By the time the divorce was finalized, Devan had aged out and Maddie was 17. Amy asked for primary custody of Maddie since Maddie's perceptions of Amy had been manipulated by the negative messages of her dad about Amy's mental health crisis. The judge was not willing to change custody because Maddie was 17 years old, even though the judge acknowledged that Maddie's dad had engaged in alienating behaviors. Amy was seeking therapy for guidance as to how to reconnect with her young adult children who were completely unresponsive to her.

Amy is the parent suffering from the highest level of hopelessness out of the three case studies presented. The divorce process was over, and while there were advantages to not being in litigation, such as less overall stress, it also meant there were no upcoming opportunities where a judge may hear the issues and make some rulings that give the parent more time with the child. Additionally, in Amy's case, one child was no longer under the supervision of the court, and the other child would soon be 18 and not required to follow a parenting plan schedule. Like Rachel, Amy will have a story to tell her therapist, and the therapist will learn who she is now, who she was in the marriage, and who she wants to be in the future. She almost had her kids to adulthood before her marriage ended, and she lived for years under the control of a demeaning partner who did not value her as a mother.

Clinicians attempting to increase hope for clients in similar situations to Amy's should offer resources such as books about parents who have reconnected with their adult children after being alienated after the divorce. These clients may need guidance and support finding ways to send loving messages on birthdays and holidays. These parents must maintain hope because they are at high risk for depression and anxiety (Harman et al., 2022). Adult children will have more freedom to reconnect with a rejected parent as their dependency on the favored parent decreases (Cartwright, 2006).

A sense of empowerment for parents in this situation will be more focused on building a fulfilling life of their own. This is similar to the work many parents must do when their children leave for college, but significantly different in terms of continued contact and future homecomings. Due to a normal developmental process, the rejected parent is not replacing day-to-day parenting duties with activities for themselves. They feel that they are doing so because their children were taken away from them; and therefore, moving on is forced instead of the natural progression of life. Processing the grief and loss associated with this experience will constitute a larger portion of the treatment plan in these cases than those parents who are just beginning the divorce process or maintaining some contact and involvement with their children.

Goal #5—Coping with Grief and Loss

In most divorces, parents experience some level of grief and loss. The very nature of divorce requires that parents will lose time with their children. Parents who were used to spending most of their time with their children will feel the loss of their presence more than those parents who traveled for work and were frequently gone. These normal and expected losses associated with divorce are compounded when children resist spending time with one of their parents. Assessment of the parent's levels of grief and loss should have occurred during the building rapport stage of the treatment. As parents shared their marital history, legal history, and the extent to which they have lost contact and connection with their child, clinicians note the types of losses reported.

The initial stages of separation and divorce are full of unknowns for the children and adults going through it. Children wonder about where the one parent will live, what their room will look like, whether they will have their favorite toys, whether they will go to the same school, how they will see their friends, and so on. Parents worry about how they will afford a separate living situation, whether they will have to get a new job, how they will survive Christmas without their children, will their children be harmed, etc. Ambiguity is difficult for people to deal with for extended periods. We seek answers that clarify what to expect when situations include unknown factors. Research has linked intolerance of uncertainty to anxiety disorders, obsessive-compulsive disorder, depression, poorer sense of well-being, and a lower ability for self-compassion (Wheaton et al., 2021; Gu et al., 2020).

Ambiguous Loss

Parents dealing with the resistance or rejection of their children are potentially dealing with high levels of anxiety. They do not know how much time they will lose with their children and have no guarantees that the resistance will decrease or how long it will take to improve. Unresolved losses are characterized by losses with no closure, no identified end, and no rituals recognizing the end of the relationship. Drawing from the research on ambiguous loss and the therapeutic concepts that have been identified for helping people grieve ambiguous loss, clinicians may be better equipped to help parents who are experiencing rejection from a child (Boss, 1999, 2006; Boss et al., 2017).

Rejected parents are often not allowed any contact with the child. When they do try to assert themselves, even in very benign ways, such as attending a basketball game, they are accused of not respecting the child's boundaries or accused of stalking behaviors. The child may attend school a few blocks from where the parent lives, may go to the neighborhood grocery store or park, and/or reside less than a mile away from a parent. Still, the parent is not allowed any contact with them, and if they happen to see them in the grocery, the child often flees in fear. It is tormenting for these parents to know that each day that goes by they are missing out on the important aspects of their children's lives.

As stated in this chapter, these parents can feel lonely and isolated. The experience of being rejected by your children is not common. These parents often suffer from embarrassment and shame as they experience implied criticism and negative judgments from friends and family who, because of their lack of understanding, think the parent must have done something wrong for the children not to want to see them. The general public and most mental health professionals have not been trained in the dynamics that can lead to resistance during the divorce process, and many find it hard to believe that a child could be manipulated by one of their parents to hate the other for unjustified reasons.

Increasing Support

Clinicians can help lessen this isolation and depression by finding ways to increase the parent's support system. One of the first ways of doing this is to connect them with people who understand what they are experiencing. Organizations such as the Parental Alienation Study Group consist of parents and professionals dealing with parental alienation. Other suggestions are offered at the end of this chapter in the section "Clinician's Toolbox." Clinicians can also decrease the parent's shame and guilt by understanding parental alienation and acknowledging the loneliness, keeping in mind that there is a fine line between empathy and pity. Empathy acknowledges the experience but does not increase feelings of victimization and helplessness.

Processing Ambiguous Losses

Boss (2006) outlines six therapeutic goals for treating ambiguous loss: (1) Finding meaning, (2) tempering mastery, (3) reconstructing identity, (4) normalizing ambivalence, (5) revising attachment, and (6) discovering hope. We will briefly discuss each of these goals here.

1. **Finding Meaning:** Finding meaning refers to a process of conceptualizing the experience that one is or has endured, no matter how nonsensical or horrific. In 1963, Victor Frankl wrote a book called *Man's Search for Meaning*. He theorized that a fundamental force in life is man's determination to make the experience or situation in which he finds himself meaningful. Frankl survived life in a Nazi concentration camp and went on to work as an existential psychologist drawing from his experience in the camp. He believed finding meaning in his experience at the time contributed to his survival and ability to move on afterward and lead a fulfilling life. Frankl found that those who lost hope in seeing a loved one were less likely to have meaning or a will to live. The clinician's task is to help clients understand where or how they derive meaning. Religious and spiritual beliefs define meaning for some, while cultural beliefs, philosophical approaches to life, and/or philanthropic and advocacy work for others.

In families where there has been severe parental alienation, an entire family system is often traumatized and grieving the loss of the child. One of the characteristics of an alienated child is the extension of the child's hatred to include all the relatives on that side of the child's family (Baker, 2007; Baker et al., 2012; Lorandos et al., 2013). Grandparents who have spent years celebrating the child, attending holiday gatherings, and going on vacations are completely cut off from any communication with the child. Therefore, the task of defining meaning may include family discussions with the therapist as the family system strives to give meaning to the child's absence in the family. As stated by Boss, "With ambiguous loss, the family's identity becomes confused because one of its members is neither in nor out of the system" (p. 76). The task of the clinician is to help the family make meaning out of their distress. While each person may have a somewhat unique experience of the loss, the family system can acknowledge individual experiences and create meaning as a family, thereby providing support for all members and potentially decreasing the sense of isolation and depression that any one member might experience.

Boss encourages clinicians to go into people's homes and listen to people in the places where they live as opposed to a clinical office. Inviting family members into the session with the parents can also be helpful when that is not possible. Clinicians working with parent-child contact problems should be prepared to work outside the normal therapeutic office environment. When parents have been estranged from their children, they need to experience each other in real-life activities. Many intensive reunification programs happen in a home-like setting where the family can bond in normal activities such as cooking a meal together or going for a hike, or in vacation-type settings that promote a feeling of fun and relaxation (Reay, 2015; Warshak, 2010). The same is true for grief work.

Clinicians can help clients find meaning by listening to their phenomenological experience of their loss, which reveals the clients' perceptions. Reality is an individual experience based on individual perceptions. Boss (2006) recommends that after the clinician understands how the client constructs reality, he/she can choose from the following actions that can help the client find meaning: "(1) naming the problem, (2) dialectical thinking, (3) religion and spirituality, (4) forgiveness, (5) small good works, (6) rituals, (7) positive attribution, (8) sacrifice for a greater good or love, (9) perceiving suffering as inevitable, and (10) hope" (p. 83).

Boss focuses on the client taking some action because she found that action was associated with resiliency. She identified four barriers to finding meaning, three of which seemed to apply to the loss of a child due to divorce: (1) hate and revenge, (2) secrets, and (3) disillusionment. When parents are so focused on their hatred of the other parent and getting revenge, they are blocking their ability to move forward, and they are not ready to find meaning and begin their journey of healing.

Keeping secrets only promotes shame and guilt. Rejected parents need to find a way to explain to people the absence of their children in their lives. Co-workers, friends, new romantic partners, and distant relatives will naturally ask where their children are. Clients need to find a basically truthful but not necessarily detailed way to explain what has happened in their family. The best answer may be that there was a divorce, and it was extremely hard on the children who felt torn between their parents. Clinicians should help parents come up with a few options for dealing with these questions. Feeling the need to keep a secret can lead to avoiding new social opportunities and building new relationships, limiting the parents' healing process.

Disillusionment refers to a process of acknowledging the trauma of what has occurred and moving into a phase of action to find new meaning. Frankl (1963) proposed three stages that a client will move through to deal with disillusionment: (1) unwillingness to acknowledge the trauma and tragedy of what has happened, (2) apathy and lack of any emotional response, and (3) an understanding that they must find a new meaning for themselves if they are going to heal. Clinicians will need to start their work with the client at whatever stage they present and then try to move them forward to a place of being able to engage in actions that help them find new meaning.

2. **Tempering Mastery:** Mastery refers to a person's belief that they have control over their life (Pearlin, 2010). Parents who raise their children with the belief that if they work hard, they can achieve whatever they want are teaching their children that they have some mastery over their own success in life. Mastery is commonly thought of as being associated with resiliency in that one's belief that they have control over their life generates beliefs that they can overcome obstacles or find creative solutions to unexpected life events that take them off course. However, Boss (2006) encourages clients dealing with ambiguous loss to temper their sense of mastery because these experiences often do not have a solution for a resolution that is guaranteed. When the situation

is impossible, the need to resolve it may decrease the person's ability to move on with their life. Boss states, "Tempering mastery means considering that much in our work, and in life, remains unknown and unresolved" (p. 107).

Therefore, clients facing absolute rejection from an adult child will need their therapists to normalize the need for mastery while also helping them learn how to live with the ambiguity of whether they will reconcile with their children. Thus, it tempers the client's need for mastery over the ultimate outcome of the relationship. The parent must find a way to accept the situation as imperfect. The clinician may need to help the parent reframe their situation - *choosing* to live with ambiguity rather than viewing oneself as helpless or a victim. Boss (2006) states that "the goal is learning to live well despite the lack of closure and imperfect absence and presence" (p. 103).

We have found it helpful to remind rejected parents who feel hopeless that the most important thing they can do for their child is to live a good life. The child needs to see a healthy parent for many reasons. They need to have a role model for what a healthy adult life looks like. Many times, the favored parent is severely compromised with mental health issues that limit their ability to have healthy relationships, professional accomplishment, and personal well-being. Additionally, children who realize that they have unjustly rejected a parent suffer from much guilt and shame for how they treated the parent (Ben-Ami & Baker, 2012). If the rejected parent has not been able to move on and is still in the depths of depression and despair, the adult child may find it too painful to return.

Moderating expectations of mastery can be aided by recognizing that things are not always fair and just (Boss, 2006). Parents who have been in custody litigation often experience the flaws and inadequacies of our judicial system, especially in its ability to manage the needs of families in crisis. Additionally, rejected parents who have lost their children due to the manipulation and brainwashing tactics of the other parent experience a deep sense of victimization at the hands of their spouse or ex-spouse. These experiences are not fair, nor are they just. The parents' ability and perhaps willingness to reconcile this will help them temper their need to right the wrong. When justice is a core value for the parent, the clinician's task is to help them find realistic and rational options that match their personality and skill set that could lead to a greater sense of justice. In situations where the child has already aged out, this might mean working with action groups to raise awareness, lobbying legislators, or helping other parents in custody litigation.

Decreasing self-blame may require that clients find an alternative narrative for why things happened the way they did that does not include blaming and shaming themselves but also does not reinforce a victim mentality (Boss, 1999). Therapists can remind these clients that they did the best they could with the knowledge they had at the time, that working with alienation is counter-intuitive, that they could not have known what they were dealing with initially, and that they did not have control over what the judge did with their case (Miller, 2018).

3. **Reconstructing Identity:** Building resiliency in the face of ambiguous loss requires the parent to find a way to expand their identity to include roles other than parent. Boss (2006) refers to this process of reconstructing identity in her writings. The clinician can help parents who have lost children to parental alienation explore questions like 'Who was I when I was parenting my child? Who am I now that my child is not living with me? Who am I now that I do not make decisions for my child? How can the role of "parent" look now versus how it used to look? Do I still want to identify as a parent? If so, how do I express that role?'

The answers to these questions are deeply personal and unique to each parent; therefore, the clinician must be patient and comfortable with ambiguity as they listen to the client grapple with all the many conflicting answers to these questions. There are cognitive and emotional changes that the client will need to make to find a new way of living that includes loss for the child who is not present and joy for their current daily experiences. Boss (2006) states that "health depends on the resiliency to be able to tolerate an identity that is not quite clear – and may never be" (pp. 116-117).

In Boss' writings, she referred to Martin Seligman's explanations of the differences between optimism and pessimism. He described pessimists as people who often interpret events as their fault, believe that the negative experience will last a long time, and believe that the event will continue to be the cause of other things that happen to them. While optimists see the event as temporary, they do not generalize the effects to other areas of their lives and attribute their inability to solve the problem to external causes beyond their control or bad luck (Boss, 1999).

Injustice may be something these parents struggle with. Clinicians working with these parents may also feel that there has been an injustice of some sort. Often, rejected parents have lost access to their children because of false allegations of abuse or distorted narratives that depicted them as incompetent parents. The client and the therapist may need to examine their worldviews regarding a just and fair world because a fundamental belief that the world is always just and always fair can create a barrier to integrating the experience in a healthy way. Reconstructing identity and grieving the loss of a child who is psychologically present but physically absent may require the parent to create a more flexible belief system that includes the possibility that bad things can happen to good people (Boss, 2019, 2006, & 2022).

Boss (1999) states that rituals like holidays, birthdays, vacations, and common family gatherings may need to be redefined in some way. Otherwise, the person experiencing ambiguous loss may avoid the activities and isolate themselves. This type of isolation will lead to depression and hopelessness and will not allow healthy resolution. She encourages therapists to use other family members to work with the client to find new ways of enjoying these activities. The family may have to decide how they define family (who is considered family) because some members may want to move forward as if the person is not living. In contrast, others will want to maintain the person as present. Everyone's perspective and emotions are valid and respected as they explore the options for moving forward.

Dialectical thinking is the ability to simultaneously hold two opposing realities as valid and real. It is "both/and" instead of "either/or." In all Boss' books (1999, 2006, 2017, 2022), dialectical thinking is discussed as integral to decreasing stress, building resiliency, and managing ambiguous loss. It pertains to the experience of rejected parents and reconstructing identity in that these parents are dealing with the situation of needing to embrace an identity that is both "parent" and "not parent." They have children out in the world and sometimes right down the street living full lives, going to school, starting college, playing basketball, getting new jobs, etc. The children's lives are often visible or known because they have social media or the events are shared by the parents of the child's friends.

When the children are still in school, the rejected parent may have options for staying involved that they will not have once the child graduates. School activity is easily obtained when the kids are in public school. However, when the child moves to college, coursework and attendance are not released to parents. This will be a loss for the rejected parent and require an adjustment in how they experience themselves as a parent. Thus, clinicians working with rejected parents may need to help these parents reconstruct their identities multiple times as the child ages and options for involvement decrease. Boss (1999) found that the greater the client's ability for dialectical thinking, the greater their resilience in constructing and reconstructing their identity in an ever-changing world. She states that "the continuity that is needed for resiliency comes from being able to live with both the absence and presence of the people close to us and in whose reflection, we come to know and re-know ourselves" (p. 142). The "Clinician's Toolbox" section at the end of this chapter contains some resources for helping clients develop dialectical thinking skills.

4. **Normalizing Ambivalence:** Normalizing ambivalence refers to acknowledging that contradicting feelings about a person and or a situation is a normal reaction to the situation. Parents who feel that they have lost a child due to the manipulations of the other parent may struggle with how to change a situation that they fear cannot be changed. They need to find a way to maintain hope in a situation where they may feel hopeless.

Resiliency and healing may come from redirecting their energy. Actions to change their own situation may be redirected to make change on a broader level or to help someone else deal with a similar situation. There is evidence in all parts of the world of parents and grandparents working tirelessly on the topic of parental alienation to change public awareness, change laws in custody litigation, and provide support. Organizations have been created that support research, education, and advocacy by parents and grandparents who have lost children due to the alienating behaviors of a previous spouse. This activity seems to help them maintain hope that their situation will change one day, but, in the meantime, they try to ensure that others will not have to endure the same trauma.

According to Boss (2006), the therapeutic goal of normalizing ambivalence is important because if feelings remain unconscious, they are destructive and interfere with resiliency and healing. Psychologists have long supported the value of being aware and acknowledging feelings. Freud (1917) long ago identified that destructive behaviors directed toward self and others can result from repressed feelings. This was expressed in his writings on defense mechanisms.

Debilitating levels of anxiety may result from unacknowledged confusion and stress as an alienated parent attempts to deal with the simultaneous loss and presence of their child(ren). It has been the authors' experience that when left unprocessed, this level of stress can interfere with the parent's ability to make decisions and take action, leading to guilt, indecisiveness, and helplessness. Somatic symptoms and depression then seep in to further inhibit the parent's feelings of hope or motivation to make productive changes for themselves, and the grief process becomes stagnant. Therefore, acknowledging that unclear and conflicting feelings are a normal part of an ambiguous situation has been helpful to many clients by creating an acceptance for feelings that could otherwise lead to destructive levels of anxiety and stress.

Boss (2007) differentiates between ambiguity and ambivalence. Ambiguity is something that is known – a situation is ambiguous. Ambivalence is an emotional state. Clinicians help their clients deal with ambiguous loss by merely naming it as such and then by freeing up their emotional and cognitive coping by normalizing the feelings of ambivalence. Alienating parents are often paralyzed by simultaneously wanting to walk away from their rejecting children and wanting to rescue them from the manipulation of the other parent. Clinicians do not need to answer which path is best – walking away or fighting. They need to help the parent continuously process the contradictory feelings so that the parent's own decision-making and coping skills are intact to help them in whatever action they need to take.

5. **Revising Attachment:** In some models of the grief cycle (Kubler-Ross, 2014), acceptance and/or closure are associated with the ability of the grieving person to move on with their life. According to Boss (2007), closure is not possible in situations of ambiguous loss. Acceptance is more about accepting that the relationship may need to be different, but the attachment to the person is still very much present.

Therefore, according to Boss' model, clinicians working with parents who are grieving the loss of a child from parental alienation should not have closure as a therapeutic goal. Instead, the goal should be to help the person revise their connection to the child and by accepting the indeterminant length of time that the child will be gone or remain distant from the parent and the reality that the child is still present in many ways. Helping these parents manage the emotional extremes of needing to cling to the child or forget the child and pretending they do not exist is one of the tasks of professionals working with this population. A healthier detachment process will include living with the ambiguity of "not needing closure but also not denying the loss" (p. 164).

Revising attachment (Boss, 2007) is a gradual, non-linear process that includes "softening" the attachment to the child, strengthening attachments to others, and building new attachments. Kubler-Ross (2014) described a five-stage linear process where one stage is resolved before the next stage is processed and experienced. Kubler-Ross' stages start with some form of denial or resistance and lead to despair and then end with acceptance. Boss (2007) stated that there is no closure and rarely acceptance for the person dealing with a situation of ambiguous loss, and therefore, the grief process needs to focus on shifting the perception of the relationship to account for the context of ambiguity.

This is definitely the case for rejected parents. Whether they are still involved in litigation or not, the hope of reconciliation will always be present in their hearts and minds. The clinician will need to allow the parent to express strong negative emotions that include self-blame, despair, guilt, shame, and rage. However, healthy resolution of these feelings requires the parent to understand they stem from a situation that appears to have no resolution, rather than meaning that the parent is inherently flawed in some way. Particularly in situations when litigation is complete, these parents can be prone to behaviors that isolate them and lead to serious levels of despair (Harman et al., 2022).

These emotions are not pathological. They are a result of the trauma of litigation, the betrayal of people they loved and were closely attached to, and the ambiguous nature of their loss. These parents will need to revise their attachment to the child and to other family members to begin creating new attachments to other people. Boss (2007) reminds clinicians that in working with situations of ambiguous loss, the goal is not to require the client to have closure, it is to help them find ways to live fulfilling and meaningful lives despite the loss.

6. **Discovering Hope:** Boss (2002, 2007) describes discovering hope as inherently connected to finding meaning. One leads to the other. Finding meaning leads to hope, and one cannot find hope without meaning. In this way, her theory for dealing with situations of ambiguous loss is circular.

Therapeutic interventions that promote hope consider the likelihood that what is hoped for will need to change over time. In the situation of a child severely affected by parental alienation, the parent's initial hopes to resolve the child's inaccurate perceptions and irrational rejection through therapeutic intervention may need to be revised. When court hearings do not provide some resolution, hopes of reconciliation through litigation may need to be revised. Therefore, hope that increases resiliency and leads to healthy adaptation is frequently changing if the ambiguous loss continues. Continuing to hold on to hope for a past situation after much time has passed without change will lead to hopelessness and limit the parent's ability to find meaning in new activities and new relationships.

Clinicians will need to help parents create new connections with other parents who have experienced the same kind of loss. Support groups are particularly beneficial when led by professionals who understand the healing component of being heard and affirmed by others who have endured the same kind of loss. Family sessions are also very valuable when extended family members are also being rejected by the child. Families can redefine hope as the divorce proceeds. These families need to express their sadness over the lost months or years of not being involved in the child's life. They have often missed out on developmental achievements that only happen once, such as graduations from middle school and high school, prom, etc. Such losses need to be expressed and future hopes defined. This is a continual process. Even when the child spontaneously returns or is required to see the family because of a new court order, the interactions may be less than fulfilling as the child learns to be in relationship with the parent and extended family after months or years of separation.

To summarize, clinicians working with this population need to be willing to be extremely patient, bear witness to a level of pain and trauma that is unlike that of normal grief and loss, help the clients reconstruct their identities and lives, and help the clients build new connections to their family members and community. The clients may need to re-evaluate their guiding principles for living life well and whether those beliefs serve them well in their current situation. What is hoped for needs to be continually reassessed and revised. The capacity to tolerate ambivalence and ambiguous situations needs to be solidified within the clinician's personality and coping skills set before they can hope to guide the client through a situation of ambiguous loss.

Goal #6—Preparing the Parent for Therapeutic Contact with the Child

When families are going through separation and divorce and a child begins to resist contact with one of their parents, legal and mental health professionals will often initially recommend family therapy. This recommendation may come when the child is still having some contact with the parent or after there has been no contact for a short or long period of time. Clinicians working with the targeted or rejected parent can help prepare the client for family therapy with the child.

One way to prepare the parent is to help the parent come up with short reflection phrases to use during the joint sessions if the child blames them for things that have happened in the past or wants to discuss all the reasons why they are mad at the parent and/or do not want to spend time with the parent. The parent is most likely aware of what the child's complaints and accusations are and, therefore, should be able to discuss them with their therapist. Targeted and rejected parents are often blamed for things they did not do, or the complaints against them are distorted to be much worse than what happened (Baker & Fine, 2008; Polak, 2020). These parents can benefit from practicing empathic responses and active listening through role-playing the comments and criticisms they expect to hear from their child.

The parent's natural response may be to debate the facts of the complaint or accusation with the child. While there may be a time when this is therapeutically necessary, it is not a productive approach in the beginning sessions of family therapy. Therefore, the parent needs to be more reflective initially, even when the statements made by the child are inaccurate. They can commit to memory some general responses that allow them to acknowledge a different version of events without sounding defensive or unwilling to hear the child out. For instance:

- Your memory of that event is different than mine.
- I look forward to talking about that with you. I did not know you perceived me that way.
- I did not know you felt that way at that time.
- I am glad you are telling me about your experience during that event. I did not realize you felt that way.

However, there are also instances when the parent engaged in hurtful behavior with the child or made a poor parenting decision. In these instances, the parent should acknowledge their behavior, apologize, and commit to finding other ways to handle their interactions with the child.

The parent may consider taking photo albums and/or videos of them and the child to share during the family session. The parent should ensure the family therapist agrees for them to do so. Photos and videos can be very helpful when much time has passed, when the child is very young, or when the child professes that they had no positive interactions with the parent. The individual clinician helping the rejected/targeted parent can help the parent choose the best photos and/or videos to take. Consultation with the family therapist is the best way to determine the type of photos and videos most helpful.

When the parent believes the other parent has bad-mouthed them, clinicians can help the parent determine the themes in the negative messages. Targeted and rejected parents want to be careful not to engage in behavior that supports these themes. There is often a morsel of truth in an alienating parent's negative messaging. For example, a common negative theme is that the parent abandoned the child. The targeted parent who has been described this way would need to be concerned about missing a scheduled appointment or not calling in to the appointment at the correct time. If the parent has been described as incompetent, the child will look for evidence of the parent doing something wrong, so being on time and prepared would be important.

Goal #7—Preparing the Parent to Receive the Child in Their Home

When a therapeutic intervention has not been successful, and courts believe that the child's rejection of the parent is unjustified, they may order that the child begin spending time regularly with the parent they are resisting or that the child spend exclusive time with the rejected parent. In either situation, the parent who has been rejected will need help preparing for the child to be in their home.

Safety Plans

Clinicians working with the rejected parent can help them prepare in several different ways. Determining the safety precautions necessary will depend on the amount of risk there is for the child to act out in a way that could harm themselves or someone else in the household.

Some parents choose to install cameras in the hallways and main living areas. This can be reassuring when there have been allegations of abuse made by the child or the other parent. Extended family members can help provide oversight if they can stay with the parent and child initially. Clinicians should help parents develop a safety plan in case of severe acting out, such as running away or self-harm. When children are much younger, severe acting out is not typically as big of a concern, and the more important preparations tend to be ensuring that the parent has the skills to manage emotions, to set a good structure for the child, to have realistic expectations of the child based on the child's age, maintain empathy for the child's positive feelings of the other parent, and engage in activities that build positive and secure attachment.

Diffusing Conflict

Psychoeducation techniques can be used to help the parent understand the futility of engaging in power struggles with the child or telling the child that their beliefs are due to the other parent alienating them. These are issues to be dealt with in therapy. Direct statements to the child that attempt to convince them that the other parent is bad or has engaged in parental alienation will only serve to intensify the need of the child to protect the other parent. The authors have found it helpful to remind parents that they are trying to build relationships with the child and that overly harsh authoritarian responses to the child's initial acting out will not help them establish a trusting relationship. They can move back into normal parental responses and discipline with time. Still, in situations where there has been significant time with no contact with the child, the parent must refrain from overreacting to rude and non-compliant behavior. The rejected parent will likely need guidance and support to differentiate between when to let something go and when to set a limit. They must focus on building positive experiences with the child and engaging in normal caretaking activities.

Conclusion

In summary, to work with a parent experiencing the rejection of their child, clinicians need to assess the level of rejection (i.e., how much contact the parent has with the child), understand the parent's previous relationship with the child, identify the child's rejecting behaviors, and help the parent find ways to maintain connection, grieve the loss, and rebuild their life. Ambiguous loss is a unique and often prolonged experience. However, the authors have observed many situations where alienated children spontaneously reunify with an alienated parent as adults. They have also had cases where a parent has parenting time but must endure rejection behaviors from a moderately alienated child for an extended period before the child can release their resistance and return to normal parent-child interactions. Many outcomes are possible, and helping these parents grieve while maintaining hope and moving on with their lives is valuable and important work.

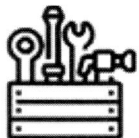

Clinician's Toolbox

- Karen Woodall Blog – https://karenwoodall.blog
- Support Group for parents of alienated children – information on Woodall's blog
- *Learn How to Talk So Children Will Listen and Listen So Children Will Talk* by Faber and Mazlish; also available in DVD teaching format
- *Positive Discipline* by Jane Nelson
- Ryan Thomas – YouTube Videos; Parent coaching
- Dialectical Thinking examples and exercises
- www.familyaccessfightingforchildrensrights.com

Chapter 10

TREATMENT WITH THE FAMILY

> **Learning Objectives:**
> 1. Understand the importance of a court order before starting treatment with the family.
> 2. Create therapeutic goals for the favored parent-child dyad.
> 3. Learn techniques to use in the favored parent-child dyad.
> 4. Create therapeutic goals for the target parent-child dyad.
> 5. Learn techniques to use in the target parent-child dyad.
> 6. Learn ways to move forward when progress stalls.

If there are parent-child contact problems, it is usually in the child's best interest to repair the issues using a coordinated family-system-based intervention. Various similar interventions are used to tackle mild to moderate cases of parent-child contact problems and the related family dynamics (Polak, 2020). While the tools and interventions may differ, a common feature is an approach that includes all family members in various combinations, where one clinician works with the entire family. Though a team approach with multiple therapists or a lead clinician might be ideal or required, this model can be more expensive and complicate the coordination of services (Fidler & Bala, 2020).

Courts ordering reunification or reintegration therapy as a part of the divorce process is relatively new (Saini et al., 2016) and often a skill set many do not learn in graduate school (Fidnick & Deutsch, 2012). Neither of the authors did, which was the impetus for this book. Working with these families can be overwhelming. While clinicians tend to want a positive rapport with their clients, sometimes half of the family system does not want to be in therapy with you in the first place (Smith, 2016)!

It is best if you do not start working with the family until you have a court order—the family needs clear boundaries and consistency to do well. You need a court order to back you up as you attempt to decrease the chaos in this family system. Each family member is struggling with intense anxiety about the situation, and the structure of the court order can serve to calm some of those anxieties. If there is a treatment team, you must communicate regularly as the family members will try to test your boundaries and triangulate. More details about how this works are covered in Chapter 11, which discusses treatment team models.

A review of the research reveals four key components essential for reunification therapy to succeed. First, you must properly assess the case (Baker et al., 2020). This usually involves, at the very least, an intake with each member of the family and getting to know where each of them is coming from, even if their complaints are exaggerated. When you start to work with this family, you have to be as neutral as possible as you work on building a relationship with each family member (Smith, 2016). You must evaluate and determine if the child's resistance is mild, moderate, or severe (see Chapter 5, "Diagnostic Considerations"). Often, you can get this information in the intakes, but sometimes, a child's resistance level can change during the therapeutic process. Sometimes, assessing the case may involve reviewing court documents or communications or talking with a professional who has more time on the case (see Chapter 3, "Assessment Procedures for Mental Health Professionals"). It is essential to review the different potential causes in Chapter 2 and keep an open mind and a willingness to be proven wrong should some contradicting evidence come your way.

Second, you must develop and monitor the treatment goals (Baker et al., 2020). This chapter describes treatment goals and techniques that can help you. New information may be obtained during your treatment that changes your conceptualization of the contact issues. Progress and regression in the contact problems may also warrant changing treatment goals.

The third component is defining treatment success and evaluating it as you work with the family. It is important to know when the family is stuck and when you may need additional assistance from the court to move forward with the family.

The fourth component is addressing the barriers to successful treatment (Baker et al., 2020). Sometimes, one part of the family keeps the rest from moving forward, and you may need to pause some parent-child sessions to work with an individual member. For instance, if the favored parent is undermining the success in the therapy room, and work with the favored parent is not improving that dynamic, then you may need to alert the treatment team or a representative of the court that you will either need further structure/intervention from the court to move forward, or you may have to withdraw from the case altogether.

THERAPEUTIC FOCI OF TREATMENT

The main purpose of reunification therapy is to improve family functioning for every family member, not just to reconnect a child with the target parent (Polak & Moran, 2017). Healthy boundaries need to be created or re-established once the family has gone through a disruption. Conflict resolution and communication skills need to improve as well as the ability to manage emotions, especially anxiety (Polak, 2020).

You will likely need to reset how the family operates at the outset. You can educate the parents that they should be equally responsible for parenting the child. At this point, it is probable that one parent will become resistant to therapy and will show signs of unwillingness to give the other parent that much authority. However, keeping the parents in the parenting role relieves the child from being caught between the two parents. The child should not feel pressured to make adult decisions and instead be allowed to be a child (Walters & Friedlander, 2010; Polak, 2020).

The parents in these families tend to use either avoidance or litigation to resolve conflicts. They typically have very little communication as they do not know how to communicate effectively in the first place (Polak, 2020). If you are able, it would be very helpful in your treatment plan to include assisting the parents in their communication, as the benefits will cascade into the entire family system.

Emotions of anxiety and loss tend to contribute to the resist-refuse dynamics in a family. It is not just the anxiety of the child at play but also the anxiety of the target parent when seeing the child. Often, there is tension and anxiety in the room when both parents are together as well, which, if the child is there, will negatively impact the child (Polak, 2020). Therefore, helping the family members manage these emotions will be an important part of your work with the family.

In working with the family system, each parent tends to want to blame the other parent as wholly responsible for the parent-child contact problems. Ultimately, that perspective is not helpful, and you may need to help the parents understand that they only have control over their own behavior. Sometimes, if they make changes to their contribution to the problem, the other parent's behaviors or attitude may change, as well as the child's behaviors. While it is true that one parent may be contributing much more to the resistance/refusal than the other parent, both parents need to be a part of the solution (Fidler & Bala, 2020).

In dealing with the resist-refuse dynamic, one of your more challenging tasks will be to manage the pace at which the sessions proceed for the child and the target parent. The favored parent will feel that you are going too fast with the resistant child, and the targeted parent will feel that you are moving too slowly. It is necessary to balance the need to make progress in reunification with the need to get the participation and support of the favored parent and the child, or you risk the parent finding a way to withdraw the child from participation (Walters & Friedlander, 2010). Some of this conundrum can be relieved by having a court order structuring the therapy and ordering participation by both parties (see Chapter 6 for an example of a formal treatment agreement).

GOALS AND TECHNIQUES

Working with the Parents

Each parent will likely blame the other parent for the family's dysfunction. Target parents will come to the office entirely blaming the other parent for alienating the child from them. While alienating behaviors may be contributing to the dynamic, identifying the case as an "alienation case" or "not an alienation case" can be too simplistic, serves to polarize the family further, and will ultimately make your job as their clinician more difficult (Fidler & Bala, 2020).

Divorce education for both parents that specifically describes alienation behaviors warns parents what not to do. Family court professionals need to be trained to learn the alienating strategies so they can better help divorced families (refer to Chapter 4 for a complete list of alienating behaviors). Furthermore, target parents need concrete suggestions on how to respond to their children exhibiting rejecting behaviors (Baker & Ben-Ami, 2011).

Goal #1–Establish Expectations for the Therapeutic Process

Early in the process, it is important to set up expectations for the reunification process so that no one is surprised. If no one has an individual therapist, and you are doing all of the work as a reunification therapist, you will have to spend some extra time building the foundation of your work. Part of this foundation is having each parent know that regular participation is required. While kids may have extracurricular activities, if they are court-ordered to do reunification therapy, it needs to be a priority for the time it is ordered. Once you are having sessions with the rejected parent-child dyad, the sessions need to be regular to make progress.

Goal #2–Establish Healthy Communication Between the Parents

Another component that needs to be addressed is parental communication. There may be a parent coach or a parent facilitator on board who is already working with the parents on that piece. If not, it may be worth your time to address it and see if you can teach the parents some basic skills. Bill Eddy's book, *BIFF for Coparent Communication: Your Guide to Difficult Texts, Emails, and Social Media Posts*, may help parents learn how to respond to each other so as not to escalate the conflict (Eddy, 2020). If communication between the parents needs more work than a few basic education sessions, you may recommend they get someone to work on that with them explicitly.

Goal #3–Establish Healthy Boundaries Between Households

Once healthier communication is established, some boundaries will be set between households. One way to help the parents establish better boundaries is to build a contract that clarifies and helps the children go from one house to another smoothly. When the children have to manage each parent's differing views on what they are allowed to bring from house to house, what they should be talking about in each house, how much information they should provide for each parent about the other parent's home, the stress the children feel starts to erode their relationships with one or both parents.

Some states have a bill of rights for children that can help in this process. You can undoubtedly adopt such a contract if your state does not have one. Texas has the Children's Bill of Rights (*Children's Rights*). These rights talk about what children of divorce can expect from their parents after a divorce. Reviewing this with each parent and having them understand what those are is helpful. If you can get them to sign off stating that they will honor their children's rights, it can be beneficial in your family therapy sessions later.

In one of the author's reunification protocols (Allen, 2023), the parent coach educates all parents on the following practices, and the parent signs a contract stating that they will adhere to them:

Parent and Family Member Pledge to Child

I will not make disparaging comments about the other parent to the child.
I will encourage a relationship between the child and the other parent.
I will not allow the child to make disparaging comments about the other parent.
I will reprimand/discipline the child for making disparaging comments about the other parent.
I will not ask the child about their therapy session or fish for information about therapy.
I will redirect the child if they begin talking with me about details of therapy.
I will not interview or interrogate the child about their time with the other parent.
I will redirect the child if they begin sharing negative things about the visit.
I will explain to the child that they need to discuss these concerns with the other parent.
I will not place the child in the middle of disagreements or conflict between parents.
I will engage in appropriate conflict resolution directly with the other parent.
I will not use the child to gain information about the other parent's life.
I will ask the other parent directly if I have questions about their life.
I will not threaten to halt therapy for the child as a form of punishment.
I will find appropriate forms of discipline that do not involve the child's therapy.
I will not discuss inappropriate topics with the child.
I will redirect the child immediately and I will ensure the child is not in hearing distance of adult conversations.
I will not guilt or shame the child for having a relationship with the other parent.
I will encourage a relationship between the child and the other parent.

I will not create scheduling conflicts to willfully interfere with therapy appointments.
I will prioritize therapy for the child, including family therapy with the other parent.
I will not undermine the parental authority of the other parent.
I will discuss differences in parenting approaches only with the other parent, not the child.
I will not encourage the child to dislike or fear the other parent.
I will encourage the child to resolve concerns with the other parent.

Working with Favored Parent-Child Dyad

When you assess the case to be in the moderate to severe range, and the child has had little to no contact with the rejected parent, there will be more preparatory work with the favored parent as well as the favored parent-child dyad needed to support the future work with the target parent and child (Walters & Friedlander, 2010).

The favored parent is usually resistant to reunification and will present as if they are really focusing on their child's needs. They will want the treatment to go slowly and for the pace to be entirely determined by the child. They will not prioritize the reunification therapy and may try to reschedule appointments due to extracurricular commitments. While you can certainly do your best to honor the child's schedule, you must also remind the favored parent that the Court needs feedback and, therefore, the reunification therapy needs to be prioritized (Smith, 2016).

Goal #1–Establish Healthy Boundaries Between Households

In families where boundaries are unclear or violated, triangulation can become a coping mechanism to deal with unresolved conflicts, and the favored parent will ally with the child against the target parent. This can be addressed by informing each family member to directly communicate with the family member they are upset with. Your task is to help the favored parent understand how they contribute to the triangulation and how it harms their child. When the child has complaints about the target parent, the favored parent is instructed not to discuss these issues with the child; instead, they should redirect the child to either the clinician or the rejected parent. The favored parent and the child should be instructed that the target parent cannot improve things if the target parent does not know how they upset the child (Smith, 2016).

When working with any dyad, it is good to set the stage that you will not talk about anyone who is NOT in the room. This will discourage disparaging the other parent (or another family member). If you used a formal agreement initially, you could refer to the treatment contract to remind the parents of the treatment expectations.

If the child is in the moderate-to-severe resistance range, you may want to confront these issues with the favored parent. If you used the Texas Children's Bill of Rights, one from another state, or your own adaptation, you could go over this in a child-friendly way in a session with both the favored parent and child. Dealing with disparaging remarks early in the process can help set the tone for future sessions.

It is helpful to preface this process by talking about how parents make mistakes and how they do not always know what they are doing after a divorce, but these are the new rules that the child's parents are going to abide by. The clinician can also acknowledge that parents may accidentally break a rule, and if the parent does break a rule, the child can either point it out to the parent or make a note of it in their head. Having them take note of it in their head decreases the chance that they will forget the infringement if they are not comfortable calling out their parent.

Another way to establish healthier boundaries is to empower the child in a healthy way. While the child should have a voice and some choices, there are some decisions that the adults should ultimately make. For instance, spending time with a parent or having a relationship with a parent is not a developmentally appropriate choice for a child to make (Smith, 2016).

Secrets and poor conflict resolution are not healthy in any relationship. Adults who have children keep secrets and reward them for reporting the "bad behavior" of another person are tacitly teaching children to lie, distort, and not deal with their relationship conflicts directly. A therapist can restate a couple of mantras in their work with the child that will help the child in their relationship with their parents as well as their other relationships:

1. Adults do not tell children to keep secrets, only surprises.
2. When you have an issue/grievance with someone, you work it out with that person rather than telling others your grievance.

Parents may need to be reminded of these rules so they can redirect the child whenever the child brings up an issue from the other household. If parents complain to the clinician about something happening in the other household, remind them how they should redirect the child and how they should know less about what is happening in the other household.

Goal #2–Favored Parent to Support the Relationship Between Child and Target Parent

Depending on how your initial sessions with the favored parent went, you may need to do additional work with the favored parent before meeting jointly with them and the child. Some favored parents can never have this session, and others struggle through it. In this session, the favored parent needs to let the child know that they want the child to have a good relationship with the target parent. Have the favored parent express to the child how important it is to have the target parent in their life. You can direct the favored parent and child to share positive things about the target parent. Take note of whether both can share positive things or if it is a struggle.

The favored parent needs to convey to the child that the child will be safe with the target parent. Some favored parents do not believe this—in those cases, you can at least have the favored parent endorse that the child will be safe in a therapy room with you and the target parent there. Ideally, the favored parent will apologize for putting the child in the middle, for saying disparaging things, and let the child know that it is not the child's fault for believing the favored parent. Do not count on an apology happening, as it is a rare phenomenon for those of us who do this work regularly.

If, in your clinical judgment, you do not think that the favored parent will be able to have this session with the child, and you think it would do more harm than good, you have a few options:

1. Choose not to have the session at all.
2. Have the session, and when the favored parent starts saying or doing something harmful, stop the session and take note.
3. Work with the favored parent to write out this information instead of risking a session where the favored parent may say things that harm the process.

The vignette below is an example of a session between the favored parent and the children that went well. These sessions take time to prepare as the favored parent is often unaware of how what they say and do impacts their children. Some favored parents can see the harm they had caused when they were struggling to manage their own hurt feelings from the divorce.

Case Vignette: Hunter, Jackson, and Maddie

Hunter and Debbie, parents of two teenagers, Maddie and Jackson, are in the earlier stages of a difficult divorce. Debbie's struggles with alcohol have created significant tensions in the family, and the kids have witnessed many loud arguments between their parents. Maddie and Jackson harbor some resentment towards their mother for her behavior while under the influence. However, their negative feelings about their mother have intensified as their dad has overshared details about the divorce, such as finances, how much she has spent on alcohol, how she has been going out behind their backs when they were married, and how she wants half of the marital assets when she is the one who ruined the marriage.

As Maddie and Jackson were refusing to see their mom at all, even after she went to an alcohol treatment program, in temporary orders, the court ordered a reunification therapist for the family. During the intake process, the clinician educated each parent on how they can keep their kids out of the middle of their conflict. Upon talking with Hunter, the clinician helped Hunter realize the impact of his oversharing. Education about the developmental needs of teenagers and understanding that he cannot treat his teenage children as his peers was provided. The actions of his wife had so hurt Hunter that he had not considered how sharing the details of the divorce may be impacting his kids. Fortunately, he did want to do what he could to repair the situation so that the divorce did not get uglier than it already was. Hunter realized that he would need his own support so he could process the upsetting details he kept learning about Debbie, so he would not attempt to process the information with his kids.

Hunter was prepared to have a session with Maddie and Jackson in hopes of helping them work on their relationship with their mom. Hunter, guided by the reunification therapist, addressed Maddie and Jackson. Hunter openly apologized for sharing too much information with them. He acknowledged that such details were inappropriate and could have made their mom look worse when she had her own hurts that the kids were not privy to. He emphasized that despite their mom's issues with alcohol, she does love them deeply. He started reminding them of ways in the past that their mom had shown her love for them. He regretted any negative influence his previous conversations might have had on their perception of her. Hunter encouraged Maddie and Jackson to rebuild their relationship with their mother.

Working with the Target Parent-Child Dyad

Target parents struggle with being patient with the reunification process. By the time they have entered reunification therapy, they may have already been without contact with their child for months or even years, so understandably, they want to move quickly and have a session with their child immediately. It is difficult for rejected parents to be patient with the process. They want the process to move quickly. Often, the rejected parent wants you to immediately correct the favored parent and call them out for their alienating behaviors. However, immediate criticism of the favored parent will not attain the best therapeutic outcomes for the family (Smith, 2016).

The rejected parents will also need some therapeutic support before engaging in the process (see Chapter 9, "Treatment with the Target Parent"). Some rejected parents have been quite traumatized and are very dysregulated and will need some therapeutic assistance before having a joint session with their child to ensure it is a productive session. One of the key jobs of the rejected parent in the joint sessions is to demonstrate that the child's narrative of that parent is incorrect. Often, that will require the parent to remain calm and regulated during the session. The rejected parent will need assistance managing his or her emotions. The rejected parent may still be grieving the loss of the marital relationship and may still be angry at the child and/or favored parent about the rejection (Walters & Friedlander, 2010).

At the beginning of the process, the child may not be willing or able to handle an in-person meeting in the therapist's office. In that case, the therapist may want first to exchange emails or video clips. The target parent may leave a meaningful gift for the child in the therapist's office. For the first live conversation, the clinician may deem it best to use Zoom, especially in cases where safety is lobbied as a primary concern. If using Zoom, the child should be in the clinician's office rather than at home with the favored parent. At some point, however, the in-person session with the child and the target parent needs to happen, and you may need to push for this session to occur (Walters & Friedlander, 2010). If the in-person session had to be somewhat forced by either you, the clinician, or the court, in order to reduce the child's distress, you may need to concede some control to the child over how such a session would occur—who sits where, who asks questions and what questions may be asked, the topics to be covered, or other issues that the child may have brought up in response to having an in-person session. You may even find it necessary to have the favored parent leave the office during the appointment.

Together, you and the child will review the child's expectations and fears about the meeting. The child typically will greatly fear the initial meeting with the rejected parent and is usually surprised that it was not as bad as they believed it would be. The rejected parent has some similar anxieties. Let the child know these feelings are common and educate them about how other child clients have managed to get through the initial meeting (Smith, 2016). Discuss what it will be like when the child and parent meet and what disappointments might be encountered (Freeman et al., 2004). Collaboratively deciding how to structure that first meeting will help reduce the child's anxiety. It may be helpful to create a secret code with the child if the child is uncomfortable and needs to speak privately during the session. This option seems to help the child even though it may never be utilized in the session.

In the first session, the parent needs to focus on child-centered goals and imagine how the child may feel. It is not unusual for both parent and child to share that they both feel anxious about this meeting. The rejected parent will need to be coached on what to expect, how to greet the child, whether a hug would be permissible, and to prepare appropriate responses to the child's resistance (Freeman et al., 2004).

Goal #1—Restore the Authority of the Target Parent

Before tackling the more challenging task of addressing past wounds or correcting misperceptions of past events, the rejected parent and child should accumulate some positive, relatively harmless, and even enjoyable experiences together (Walters & Friedlander, 2010). While the initial session with the target parent may be guided mainly by the child's preferences to reduce distress, eventually, the authority of the rejected parent needs to be restored. Maybe the child offers a few activities for the session, and the rejected parent gets to choose which one they do. You may also give the target parent choices on what to work on that day, and then the parent makes the choice. Sometimes, the child will demonstrate disappointment in the parent's choice; the target parent may need some preparation before the joint session to manage the disappointment in a manner that does not undermine their authority.

Goal #2—Address Real Relationship Obstacles

Sometimes, the child wants to unload all their complaints about the rejected parent in one of the first sessions. Such a session can be very difficult emotionally for a target parent, and the parent may need some coaching and support beforehand. It is imperative that the rejected parent respond empathetically to the child's complaints without admitting to anything that the parent did not do.

When a child comes to a parent with an accusation, Baker and Fine (2008) recommend the following steps:

1. Show appreciation and gratitude that the child has brought it up to you—not anger or defensiveness. "Thank you for letting me know why you have been so upset. I know that must have been hard for you to share with me."
2. Show compassion and understanding. "I can tell you are really angry about this."
3. Show empathy by putting yourself in your child's shoes. "If I were you and thought my dad did X, I would be furious, too."
4. Make a one-sentence explanation of what happened. If it is false with no truth, you can say, "That didn't happen." If it is a subjective experience, you can say, "I do not see it the same way."
5. Return to gratitude and compassion.

Since the rejected parent is imperfect, the child likely has some genuine issues they must address. Maybe the target parent is loud when they are angry about something. It is important that the target parent listen to the child's concerns, acknowledge what they have done that may have hurt the relationship, and then apologize and talk about how they can perhaps work towards altering the harmful behavior in the future. The child's expectations should also be discussed, as it is unrealistic for the child to expect a parent's long-term behaviors to be fixed entirely immediately.

If the child has complaints against other family members, such as a grandparent, aunt, or uncle, you may also choose to include them in a session. Sometimes, the child has overheard negative statements about the favored parent by the rejected parent's family, and the child is upset about that. The child's feelings about such hurtful behaviors need to be acknowledged.

Target parents may get upset at the "unfairness" of it all at first. It seems that the favored parent can do so many things that the rejected parent cannot get away with doing. It is often the case that the child has much more forgiveness and tolerance for the failures of the favored parent, even to the point that the child does not seem to perceive these failures. You will need to remind the target parent that while it may not be fair at this point in their relationship, the target parent pointing out the unfairness to the child will not help them to move forward in their relationship with their child. They will need to process the unfairness of the situation in an individual session, not one with the child.

Goal #3—Correctively Re-Experience the Family

Sometimes, the child wants to start the process by addressing the issues they have with their target parent right away; sometimes, the child is uncomfortable with going in headfirst, so to speak, and would prefer a lighter session that may just have some basic conversation or a game. You and the child can decide what that would look like. If light conversation is desired, all kinds of conversational cards can be used for such a session, but there are other options as well.

One barrier that often arises during the reunification process is the different viewpoints on key events. Before going into these difficult discussions, it would be helpful for you to point out that it will be challenging to decide what happened, and they will have different perspectives, especially as it is an emotionally difficult event for each of them. The pre-education before the problematic conversation is hoped to help temper the emotions. First, allow the child to describe their perception of the key incident involving the rejected parent. Then, get permission from the child to have the target parent report their perception of the same incident. Sometimes, the child will become very upset and agitated at the parent's re-telling. Validate the child's frustration while, at the same time, discussing how now that they are in therapy when other such challenging events occur, they will be able to discuss them more timelier. Sometimes, the only accomplishment of such a session is for the child and rejected parent to acknowledge the hurt and pain caused by the incident and to apologize (Smith, 2016).

When you get the child and target parent in the room (or via electronic face-to-face contact), you may very well see some of the child's once-hidden enjoyment of their rejected parent. Having the target parent come prepared with old pictures, videos, and proof of positive experiences between them and the child can help bring about the memories the child has attempted to suppress. Talking about these old memories can help bring about those positive feelings toward a rejected parent (Harman et al., 2021).

Progress in sessions between the target parent and the child may be followed by regression. It could be due to the child's fear of the unknown. It could be due to the favored parent discovering how positive the session was and subsequently reacting negatively with the child. While you may not be privy to what is happening after everyone leaves your therapy office, you will notice regression in this process. You will need to handle it, sometimes by pointing out the discrepant behaviors and wondering aloud what has changed. For example, you may say, "Last time you were here, you left here excited about what we were going to do today. Today, you came here acting like you did not want to be here. I wonder what has happened in between sessions to change how you feel about things?" You may not get an answer to this from the child, and it would not be a bad idea to let that statement hang there for a bit before moving forward with what you were planning to do in the session. Sometimes, just pointing out the discrepancies in the child's behavior can prompt the child to change their attitude for the better. Your job as a clinician at this point is to try to stop the regression and to keep moving the family in a forward direction once again (Smith, 2016).

To correctively re-experience the family, it can be helpful for the rejected parent to bring in videos and photographs of their lives together before the contact disruption. If the child seems to still be in a place where they may be upset by more recent events, the parent may want to start when the child was just born. It can be very helpful if the target parent can recount the positive memories with the favored parent at the beginning of their lives together. Knowing that his parents loved each other at one point can help open the child's perspective to other positives of the rejected parent. Since the child's infancy is not a part of the life they remember, the target parent can talk about this event positively without much arguing or remembering things differently. While the child may have heard opposing perspectives from their favored parent, the rejected parent can gently reply, "I just remember it differently." It is imperative that the target parent not take this opportunity as one to argue with the favored parent through the child. Instead, it is a time for the parent to discuss fond memories.

Another challenge that may arise in family therapy when trying to re-experience the family correctively is addressing the child's cognitive distortions. While the child may have covered the basics of cognitive distortions in individual therapy, these distortions may still need to be revisited within the family context. Children who reject a parent often express their concerns using strong, extreme language and labels. You need to ask the child for specific details and examples of what actions have led them to perceive the parent's behaviors as negative. Through this process, the child may realize that the evidence they used to form their conclusions is limited or at least open to different interpretations. This exercise helps children learn the value of avoiding exaggerated language and jumping to conclusions. Instead, it encourages them to use concrete details and flexible thinking when expressing their concerns (Smith, 2016).

Considerations with Siblings

Siblings often respond to parental conflict in ways that reflect their unique personalities, genders, and developmental stages. Each child in the family may also experience the conflict differently, influenced by how the parents communicate with them individually. For instance, one sibling may internalize the conflict more, while another may express it outwardly, perhaps through rebellion. Meanwhile, another sibling might attempt to distance themselves from the conflict entirely, acting as it doesn't affect them. These varied responses also extend to their relationships with the targeted parent, as each sibling may relate to or view this parent in distinct ways. Each child should be encouraged to distinguish thoughts of their own versus those of their siblings (Walters & Friedlander, 2010).

Given these dynamics, it is generally advisable for therapy involving the targeted parent to occur with one sibling at a time. Family therapy with all siblings present risks the siblings forming a united front against the targeted parent, leading to groupthink and increased hostility. In such a setting, the likelihood of any sibling expressing positive feelings towards the alienated parent decreases, as they may fear that any display of affection will be reported back to the favored parent, potentially leading to negative consequences. Therefore, the target parent should only do family therapy sessions with one sibling at a time to create a safe space for each sibling to explore their true feelings without the influence of the other siblings or the fear of retaliation from the favored parent. This approach allows for more authentic communication between the targeted parent and each child.

Case Vignette: Debbie and Maddie

In her one-on-one session with Debbie, Maddie confronted her mother about the chaos caused by her drinking. She described in detail many instances where her mother's drinking caused embarrassing situations and instances where Maddie did not feel safe in her own home. Debbie acknowledged her past behavior and apologized, demonstrating her willingness to change and rebuild their relationship. Maddie and her mom decided they would talk more as other memories came up for Maddie, but Maddie wanted to move forward as she had really missed time with her mom. Her mom's apology felt sincere enough to Maddie that she was comfortable setting up a time to have lunch with her mom that week.

Case Vignette: Debbie and Jackson

Jackson's session with Debbie was much more challenging. Jackson's deep-seated anger and detailed recounting of his mother's past mistakes underscored how much negative impact his mother's actions had on him. Debbie maintained her calm and open stance and acknowledged how she had hurt Jackson and their family. Her empathetic apologies helped Jackson de-escalate in the session, and he left the session somewhat calmer. While he did not seem ready to spend any unstructured time with his mom, he was willing to come to future sessions to work on things with his mom.

Maddie and Jackson's differing responses to their mom in a therapy session highlight how each relationship is unique and will require different interactions to heal. Jackson is going to need more time and attention to deal with past hurts before he can move forward with his mom.

RECOMMENDATIONS WHEN PROGRESS STALLS

When progress stalls in family therapy, it is often a sign that the current therapeutic strategies need to be readjusted. You may begin by just taking a step back to review the therapy process up to when progress slowed. First, make sure your therapy goals are still relevant. Are there new goals that need to be added to address new issues that may have surfaced? Have some goals been accomplished?

Also, start looking at each family member individually, perhaps even asking each one for their perspective about what is helping in therapy and what is not. Evaluate the interpersonal dynamics between different family members that may be creating obstacles. Individual sessions with each client may help you understand if unresolved issues need to be addressed before moving forward with the family as a whole. You may need to have a session with two of the siblings before moving forward. Sometimes, the parents may need some work to de-escalate their conflict before you can proceed.

If one or more family members become uncooperative, it may be beyond your ability to work effectively with the family. If you have releases to contact attorneys, it would be wise to let each attorney know the status, and if they have a client who is not cooperating, they need to know that as well. Sometimes, attorneys are the therapist's best ally and can be integral to leading the family to a new path forward. On the other hand, if you have one attorney who is blind to the faults of their client and is too invested in defending their client rather than moving the family forward, a treatment team meeting with both attorneys present may be the best way to proceed. This may result in a court hearing where you present your findings. This is where the mental health/legal system interlock can be especially helpful in creating meaningful interventions if the court orders them. If orders are not made that help remove the barriers currently blocking the progress in family therapy, the court may decide to leave the family system as it is, but you, as a clinician, have done what you can to help. Even if you feel like your clinical work did not succeed as you had wished, know that it could be that your work with the family may have planted some seeds that will later come to fruition.

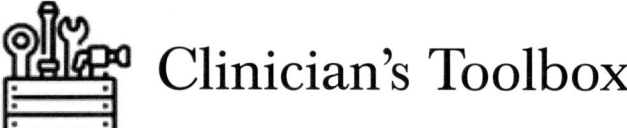

Clinician's Toolbox

- ✗ *BIFF for Coparent Communication: Your Guide to Difficult Texts, Emails, and Social Media Posts* by Eddy, Burns, and Chafin
- ✗ *Texas Children's Bill of Rights*
- ✗ Activities:
  - Conversation Cards
  - Family photos

Chapter 11

TREATMENT TEAM MODELS OF INTERVENTION FOR SEVERE CASES OF PARENTAL ALIENATION

> **Learning Objectives:**
> 1. Understand the differences between treatment for severe parental alienation and milder levels of resistance.
> 2. Be able to identify the intensive treatment programs available that have peer-reviewed outcome research.
> 3. Understand the components of a team approach to working with parent-child contact problems.
> 4. Know the skills needed for a team leader and the duties they perform.

The purpose of this chapter is to explore treatment interventions for severely alienated children, understand the components of a team approach to working with families affected by moderate to severe alienation, and understand the duties and purpose of the team lead role.

As a reminder, severe cases are identified primarily by the child's entrenched rejection and expressed hatred for one parent, which is unjustified or unsupported by the reasons for the hatred and the facts in the case (Bernet et al., 2018; Warshak, 2018; Gardner, 1985). These children express extremely polarized views of their parents (Warshak, 2013), demonstrated in objective measures such as the Parental Acceptance and Rejection Questionnaire (Bernet et al., 2019). Their all-negative view and complete rejection of the parent differentiates them from children who are estranged from a parent for bona fide abuse and maltreatment (Bernet et al., 2020). These children have been described as the hardest to work with by treatment providers specializing in contact refusal. It is not unusual for these kids to make extreme threats to harm or kill themselves or the parent, run away, or burn the parent's house down if they are forced to spend time with the parent (Warshak, 2010 & 2013; Reay, 2015; Gardner, 2001). While there are some recommendations for providers working in an outpatient setting with these children and their parents (see Chapters 7, 8, and 9), there is a general consensus in the research that providing individual, outpatient treatment while the child remains living primarily with the alienating parent is not productive and can be harmful (Warshak, 2020; Dunne & Hedrick, 1994; Baker et al., 2020). There are three treatment programs for severely alienated children that have documented outcome research demonstrating them to be safe and effective. The authors acknowledge that other programs may be available for these families but wanted to focus only on the programs that have provided outcome research in peer-reviewed journals.

Family Bridges

The Family Bridges program is a four-day intensive. In most cases a court has ordered that the child(ren) and the rejected parent attend the program together because of findings that the child is irrationally rejecting the parent and that the favored parent has been primarily responsible for the child's rejection of the parent.

The Family Bridges program requires a specific court order that places the child in the exclusive custody of the rejected parent for at least 90 days. Ideally, the child and the rejected parent begin the program as soon as court proceedings have ended. When there are concerns about the child being transported by the rejected parent to the program site, a private transportation company may be used to chaperone and deliver the child to the program site.

Two trained facilitators are used for each intensive, and at times, there may be a third professional present, taking notes and shadowing the other facilitators. Family Bridges facilitators are usually mental health providers selected by Family Bridges to receive specialized training in the philosophy and program principles. The professionals invited to receive training have usually already exhibited competence and expertise working with children affected by severe parental alienation.

Hence, the additional training in the Family Bridges protocol creates a highly specialized and expert treatment team.

The curriculum for Family Bridges evolved from programming developed by Dr. Randy Rand for the Center for Missing and Exploited Children to help children and parents reunify after being separated due to abduction. Abducted children are often brainwashed by their abductors to believe the missing parent is dangerous and abusive. Some of these children may have been missing for years and not remember the parent they are being returned to. The program was designed to bring relief to these traumatized children as quickly as possible (Warshak, 2010). It made sense that these same treatment principles could be applied when working with irrational rejection since it is often based primarily on false beliefs, opinions, and perspectives instilled in the child by the favored parent.

The goals of the program are to (1) help children adhere to court orders that essentially change their primary custody to the rejected parent and restrict their contact with the favored parent and (2) to improve the relationship between the child and the rejected parent (Warshak, 2018). Other programming goals/objectives include strengthening the child's critical thinking skills, strengthening the parent's ability to parent with empathy and also set healthy limits, increase the child's ability to have realistic views of both their parents, and teach the children how to stay out of their parents' conflict (Warshak, 2010).

The programming content is delivered in a more educational and experiential style than a traditional therapeutic style. Concepts are taught from areas such as psychology, sociology, cognition and memory, and neuroscience. The course work resembles that taught in psychology programs and is adapted to the child's developmental stage. In this way, the program relieves the children of needing to place blame or choose one parent over the other. The participants receive information that allows them to generalize those concepts to their own experiences without having to acknowledge the failures and mistakes of their own or their parents (Warshak, 2013).

While the rejected parent and the child attend the four-day treatment program and then spend at least the next two to three months together, the favored parent begins treatment with a Family Bridge's after-care specialist. This work aims to learn how they negatively impacted the child's relationship with the other parent and to make behavioral changes that will decrease the likelihood that they will continue to engage in alienating behaviors. Resuming contact between the child and favored parent depends on the favored parent completing their part of the program, demonstrating insight about their contributions to the problems, and committing to discontinuing the alienating behaviors.

The following characteristics are exhibited by children appropriate for referral to the program and were taken from the Family Bridges website (www.buildingfamilybridges.com):

1. A child's view of a parent and other relatives is unrealistic.
2. The child refuses contact with a parent or shows extreme reluctance to spend time with that parent.
3. The family needs help adjusting to court orders that place the child in the sole custody of the rejected parent and suspend contact between the child and the other parent until specified conditions are met.
4. The child's negative attitudes and behavior toward the parent are not a reasonable and proportionate response to that parent's behavior toward the child.

Rejection of a parent for the following reasons would NOT support a referral to Family Bridges (Warshak, 2010):

1. Children's whose rejection is reasonable and proportionate.
2. Families in which the court finds that a child's relationship with a rejected parent is severely damaged but that it is in the child's best interest to remain with the favored parent.
3. Families in which children who reject a parent spend most of their time away from that parent, or who will be with the rejected parent only for a short period of time before returning to the favored parent (i.e., the court was not in favor of allowing the child extended exclusive time with the rejected parent) (p. 56).

There have been two outcome studies completed on Family Bridges by Richard Warshak. The first, in 2010, consisted of 12 families and 23 children. The second, in 2018, consisted of 52 families and 83 children. The 2010 outcome research found that 22 of the 23 children experienced a successful reunification with the formerly rejected parent and that 18 maintained that positive relationship 2-4 years later. The 2018 outcomes documented that 61 of the

83 kids reported an improved relationship with the parent at the end of the Family Bridges workshop, and 67 of 68 parents reported an improved relationship with their child at the end of the workshop. The participants also reported positive experiences in the workshop and felt they were treated with respect and kindness. The children were observed to be much more cooperative after the workshop than they were at the outset.

Turning Points for Families

Turning Points for Families (TPFF) was developed by Linda Gottlieb, as a four-day intervention for severely alienated children and their rejected parents. It is described on her website (turningpointsforfamilies.com) as a "therapeutic vacation" and a "transitional intervention to jump-start the healing of a severed or severely damaged relationship between a child and a fit parent..." Like Family Bridges, Gottlieb specifies that the program is unsuited for children rejecting a parent for legitimate reasons. Also, like Family Bridges, TPFF requires that contact between the favored parent and the child be suspended for at least 90 days to give the rejected parent and the child time to receive treatment and recover their original attachment and give the favored parent time to learn how their behavior negatively impacted the child's relationship with the other parent.

The program content for TPFF is based on Salvador Minuchin's structural family therapy principles, which state that change is most likely to occur when people change for those they love and whom they feel love them. The content is described as "a symbolic-experiential intervention." Unlike Family Bridges, the content combines family systems therapy with psycho-educational techniques. Each day of the four-day intervention begins with a therapeutic/educational component, which lasts 3-4 hours. This is followed by experiential activities where the parent and child choose activities to enjoy together and are accompanied by the program facilitator. Examples of activities are visiting museums, swimming, ice skating, hiking, etc. Afterwards, the parent and child have dinner and evening activities on their own and the program facilitator remains on call.

Aftercare is usually established by working collaboratively with a local family therapist. At the end of the no-contact period, a report is issued outlining the progress of the family members, recommending future treatment needs, and stating whether it is in the child's best interest for contact with the favored parent to resume.

In 2021, Harman et al. conducted a program evaluation of TPFF. The evaluation examined two primary questions: (1) Was TPFF effective – did the relationship between the parent and the child improve, and (2) Was TPFF safe – did children experience any harmful effects by participating in the program? Fifty-two children from thirty families were evaluated. Most of the children had been separated from the parent for, on average, 2-4 years. The evaluators reviewed court documents related to each family. They found that the children were often described as threatening to run away, to self-harm, and run away from law enforcement if they were forced to see the parent, and yet, all but two of the children traveled with the rejected parent to the program site in New York without incident.

The results of the evaluation provided evidence that the children who attended TPFF were safe. The children did not engage in self-harm or attempt to run away prior to the program starting, during the program or after the program was completed. Consistent and positive ratings by the family members on communication, cooperation, and emotional support showed that the relationships between the parent and the child improved because of participation in the program.

The Family Reflections Reunification Program (FRRP)

FRRP was developed by Kathleen Reay in 2012 after years of professional experience serving as a custody evaluator and family therapist working with families going through high-conflict separation and divorce. The model she designed was based on two existing programs at the time, Family Bridges and Overcoming Barriers. The main objective was to reunify severely alienated children with their rejected parents. As with the other two programs described in this chapter, FRRP is not appropriate for children who refuse contact with a parent for justified reasons such as abuse, neglect, or exposure to domestic violence. The program targeted children between the ages of 8-18, from high-conflict families (Reay, 2015).

Like Gottlieb's Turning Point for Families program, FRRP also works from a family-systems perspective. The program attempts to include the favored parent as well as siblings and extended family members in the intervention. FRRP has the following program goals (Reay, 2015):

1. Healthy adjustment in the child.
2. Increase the child's ability and capacity for critical thinking.
3. Increase the child's awareness about how they became alienated.
4. Increase the favored parent's awareness about how the child became alienated.
5. Improve the boundaries between family members (parent to parent and parent to child) and create a healthy family structure so that parents are in appropriate parenting roles and children are acting as children.
6. Improve the co-parenting skills between the parents for communication and negotiation and problem-solving on matters related to the child.
7. Keep the reunification stable and consistent over time.
8. Enhance the child's relationship with both parents unless there are safety concerns for the child with one parent.

The program requires that the participants travel to the program site and stay at the site for the duration of the intervention. The child begins with psychoeducation without any involvement with the rejected parent. The rejected parent arrives after the child has started the initial phase of treatment and begins working with a therapist on their own to prepare for a meeting with the child. Next, the parent and child begin working on activities together and spending time in experiential outdoor activities. After successfully spending time together, the parent and child move to shared living quarters and enjoy a celebration planned by the child, which marks the end of their treatment and successful reunification.

During this time, the favored parent receives treatment from a provider trained in the FRRP model. They may receive treatment in their own community when there is a locally trained clinician, or they may do so virtually or at a site close to the location of the program intervention. An aftercare plan is created before the child and the rejected parent leaves the facility. It may include continued therapy with an FRRP-trained clinician.

The court usually refers families to the program. A court order suspending contact between the favored parent and the child is required. It usually includes a change in child custody from the favored parent to the rejected parent. The favored parent's time with the child is reinstated as they show insight into their own contributions to the child's rejection of the other parent and the capacity to change their behavior.

Dr. Reay published outcome data on 12 families and 22 children in 2015. Her program demonstrated a 95% success rate, with 21 of the 22 children able to reunify with their rejected parents. Successful reunification was quantified by the quality of parent-child interactions, the amount of shared positive activities, and the quality of their conversations and statements to each other. The one child that did not reunify left the intervention early because the favored parent was diagnosed with a terminal illness at the onset of the intervention.

The families were followed for one year after their participation in the program. All 21 children maintained positive attachments with their once-rejected parents, and most of the favored parents made significant progress. Other program findings were (1) the children were not harmed or traumatized by being removed from their favored parent, (2) a temporary or permanent reversal of custody combined with restricting time with the favored parent was beneficial, and (3) the child demonstrated a renewal of their original positive attachment and relationship with the rejected parent (Reay, 2015).

FRRP was not operational for several years due to Dr. Reay's inability to facilitate the program. However, at the time of writing this chapter, the authors were aware that Dr. Reay was beginning to accept families for the program again and thought it important to include this as one option for severely alienated children. The authors suggest that those interested contact Dr. Reay through her website, listed in the "Clinician's Toolbox" section of this chapter, for more information about the program and referral process.

All three programs listed require that the court suspend contact between the child and the favored parent, and all three require a court to order the child's participation in the program. Each program may have its own preferred court order language. Clinicians who are not having success in treating children who reject contact with one parent unjustifiably may recommend that parents and lawyers research these programs as the next higher level of care.

Therapeutic Treatment Teams

In this section of the chapter, the authors describe the concept of treatment teams and review some of the literature on their structure and composition, the benefits and pitfalls of using treatment teams, and the role of the team leader. Treatment teams working with high-conflict families may consist of various professionals helping the family, such as individual and family therapists, coparenting counselors/coaches, parent educators, psychiatrists, medical professionals, and educational professionals. An additional neutral professional who does not directly provide mental health services but understands the treatment needs of these families may serve as the treatment team lead. Treatment teams have been described in the literature as a potentially effective way to manage high-conflict families where a child resists contact with a parent (Walters & Friedlander, 2010; Sullivan, 2019; Friedlander & Walters, 2016; Johnston et al., 2001).

Practitioners working with high-conflict families understand that each person has their own contributions to the problems, albeit some family members may contribute much more than others. Changes to the family system often require each member to address their contributing behavior and beliefs, which can require professionals with different expertise. For instance, a parent suffering from a mood disorder may need the assistance of a psychiatrist. In contrast, problems in the relationship with the child may require the specialization of a family therapist.

In high-conflict families where the child is resisting contact with one parent, there could be both negative influence from the favored parent and overly harsh and critical parenting from the rejected parent contributing to the child's rejection. In such a case, the parent-child contact problem may need to be addressed with several different interventions like parenting education for the rejected parent, family therapy for the parents and the child, and psychoeducational techniques for the favored parent to understand how their behavior is bolstering the child's refusal to see the other parent (Johnston & Campbell, 1988; Fidler et al., 2013; Judge & Deutsch, 2017).

In their 2016 article, Walters and Friedlander discuss the difficulties in dealing with intractable resistance in a child, which they differentiate from milder forms of resistance during divorce and separation. They offer guidelines for professionals working with this severe level of resistance that include using a team of professionals, having specific court orders, and mental health and legal professionals working collaboratively.

Their recommendations for successful intervention reflect much of the authors' experiences in working with cases of severe rejection:

(1) The court order and oversight from the court work to contain the family which consists of some members who are fundamentally opposed to change, (2) collaboration of professionals with specialized knowledge working in alignment with each other, and (3) the work is often non-traditional in nature and does not follow traditional methods of therapy.

Johnston and colleagues (2001) proposed a model called Multi-Modal Family Intervention (MMFI) to treat families when a child was resisting contact with a parent during separation and divorce. They further refined the model ten years later (Friedlander & Walters, 2010). The treatment goals for MMFI were broader than those for outpatient "reunification" therapy. In addition to resolving the child's resistance to the parent, they sought to address the impact of the separation/divorce on the child, increase the child's coping mechanisms, address the child's distorted thinking, address the child's psychological splitting (all good and all bad views of their parents), and improve co-parenting with healthy parent to parent and parent to child boundaries and communication.

Treatment teams can be large or small. Walters and Friedlander (2016) define a small team as consisting of one mental health professional – the family therapist and one legal professional and one professional to interface with the legal professionals and provide oversight and accountability. The large team model consists of several mental health professionals – individual counselors for children and parents, a family counselor, parent educators, and multiple legal representatives, as well as one professional that interfaces between the MHPs, the legal professionals, and the court to provide oversight and hold family members accountable.

We have been involved in a small team approach and a large team approach. We have also implemented the small team approach ourselves with one serving as the team leader and one serving as the family therapist. We have found that small teams have benefits in terms of the intervention staying streamlined, treatment goals being easily adjusted, and changes to the communication and contact between the parents and the children being implemented quickly.

The larger the team, the harder it is to keep all professionals working in unison. One of the most common failures of the team approach is the tendency for individual team members to become advocates for their client's narrative and depart from a unified approach to helping the family (Sullivan, 2019). One common dynamic from our perspective is an individual therapist who believes their client's narrative that the other parent is abusive and harmful to the children, thereby supporting the child's resistance to the parent and maintaining that the child should have no contact even though the evidence does not support it and/or that the court found otherwise.

Collaborative teams do not run themselves. They need a leader who oversees managing the case, coordinates team meetings, communicates regularly to the attorneys about the status (progress or lack of progress), and provides testimony at status hearings. The team leader needs to have extensive knowledge and experience in providing interventions to ensure appropriate treatment goals and recognize when the treatment needs to be adjusted. The team leader is not in a therapeutic role. They do not deliver clinical services; however, a successful team intervention relies on the wisdom and skill of a leader who has provided clinical services to this population and recognizes the need for changes to the intervention and parent-child contact.

The court order should give the team leader some authority to change parenting time schedules and select or change mental health providers if new services are warranted. If one parent disagrees with the recommendations, they can request a court hearing, and the judge will rule on whether the recommendations should be implemented. In Texas, where the authors are licensed, the team lead role is best suited for guardian ad litem (GAL) because the Texas Family Code allows GALs to make possession and access recommendations. Other states may have court designations such as a parenting coordinator, special master, or case manager that accommodate the needs of this role.

One example of how the team lead's authority to choose treatment providers can be helpful is a case where the child's therapist determines that the child is suffering from an anxiety disorder and thinks that it is so severe that it exasperates the contact issues with the parent. The clinician recommends to the team that the child be assessed by a psychiatrist for medication. The team leader can help the parents select the provider and recommend that the child be seen within a specific time period. Without this authority, conflict and disagreement between the parents about whether the child should be assessed and/or who the child should see would stall progress in the reunification.

Another example that is much more delicate to address but happens regularly is a situation where an individual therapist has been working with the child or the favored parent prior to the court implementing a team approach. The clinician has supported the child's refusal to see the parent and does not believe the child should be forced to see the parent if they do not want to. This type of treatment is not conducive to the treatment team's goal of resolving the child's refusal so that the parent and the child can enjoy a good relationship and spend time together. When the treatment team lead is given the authority to choose and change the providers, the lead can replace a clinician who has taken on a role of supporting the parent or the child's unjustified refusal to see the other parent with one who is willing and able to meet the court's goal of reunification.

Confidentiality should be addressed in the court order or the legal documents developed by the attorneys that allow all the MHPs to share information between themselves and with the team lead. The orders should also state clearly that the goal of the intervention team is to resolve the parent-child contact problems and re-establish parenting time at a rate consistent with the rejected parent's parenting capacity.

We have found it extremely helpful for the court to schedule regular 30- to 60-day review hearings once they order an intervention for the family. When lawyers are defining the terms of the intervention and the order without a hearing, they should also schedule review meetings between themselves and the team lead. This is helpful in several ways. The family members will more likely comply with the requirements of treatment when they know that an authority will frequently assess their participation. The treatment team will be able to make changes to the plan and the parenting time schedules more quickly if they need to request those changes from the judge. When one parent opposes the recommendations, which happens frequently, a judge will be the decision maker. And finally, any problem that is holding up progress can be resolved promptly with changes to the court order. When everyone is abiding by the intervention plan and following the recommendations of the team lead, a status hearing can be passed.

The authors compose their team reports to the court and lawyers in a consistent format and aim to have them submitted to the court and the attorneys within seven days of the status hearing or review meeting. The report contains the dates of all the team meetings and all the therapeutic appointments that the family has had since the last hearing. It describes the progress that has been made, challenges and impediments to progress, and includes recommendations for additional services and increased or decreased contact between the children and the parents.

As the treatment advances and if it is working, the "progress" section should become much longer than the "challenges and impediments to progress" section. Seeing this change is particularly useful in determining whether the intervention is working. It also becomes apparent if one parent's behavior consistently causes problems and is resistant to change because it consistently shows up in the "impediments to progress section." When outpatient services are not creating a change in the level of resistance in the child or in a parent's destructive influence, a change to the parenting time schedules or custody may be necessary. The court appreciates the documentation in these reports that supports such a serious ruling.

The treatment team members do not always agree on whether parenting time schedules should be changed or whether there should be a custody change and a suspension of the child's time with one parent. In this case, the team lead assesses all the opinions of the providers and makes the final decision. The authors include such dissension in the write-up to the court so that the court is aware that some of the team members disagreed. The team leader should explain why their decision differs and then support that decision.

Clinicians cannot make custody decisions without completing a custody evaluation, so ultimately, that decision could not fall to them. This represents another valuable aspect of the team lead role. Interventions aimed at reducing a child's resistance to a parent and increasing parent-child contact will necessitate changes to the parenting time schedules.

Another benefit to this design is that the team lead role creates a buffer between the legal activity in the case and the mental health professionals (MHP). We have found that most MHPs are relieved by not having to appear at court hearings or make time in their schedules to report to two or three different lawyers for one case. It has been our experience that this approach has relieved much of the burden from individual MHPs having to be present at all the hearings.

The team structure can also address some of the risk-management issues related to working with this population (Warshak, 2020; Sullivan, 2019), not to mention provide support for the many stresses related to working with these contentious families. Regular team meetings allow clinicians to discuss their treatment techniques and goals with other professionals and receive supportive and critical feedback.

Other areas of this book have discussed potential problems for clinicians working individually with only one family member during a custody dispute. The possibility of children and parents telling individual therapists what they want them to believe rather than what is true can be managed by team meetings where other professionals share their information about the family. The team structure allows for some fact-checking as MHPs working with other family members offer another perspective and provide additional facts to which the individual clinician would otherwise not have access.

Children's comments are particularly susceptible to the influence of parents' underlying agendas to retain more custody. The child's clinician should remain astute to the possible explanations of why the child reports certain events and how they describe their own behaviors during those events. For example, in parent-child contact situations, there are often reports made by children describing distress when transitioning to the other parent. In a team meeting, the clinician working with the parent receiving the child can report whether they have heard a similar or quite different description of the child at transition time. This increases the likelihood that the child's therapist is working with accurate information.

The team leader continually assesses whether the parent-child contact issues are improving and suggests changes in the approach when they are not. The team leader is also responsible for confronting clinicians who do not remain objective, are not using the recommended approaches for court-involved therapy, and do not appear to have adequate specialized training working with families in litigation. This oversight can potentially reduce the likelihood that clinicians will receive board complaints for working in an area without specialized training, working in a way that further entrenches the child's resistance, or not referring the child or family to a different mode of intervention or higher level of care.

Highly contentious families where moderate to severe parental alienation has occurred and the child's refusal toward a parent is entrenched may require specialized interventions. Treatment teams can be a resource for managing the varied professionals needed to address the family's needs. For multiple providers to be organized to help the family, the authors have found it necessary to have one person designated as a "team lead." The lead should be an expert in parent-child contact problems and parental alienation and serve as a bridge between the mental health professionals and the legal professionals.

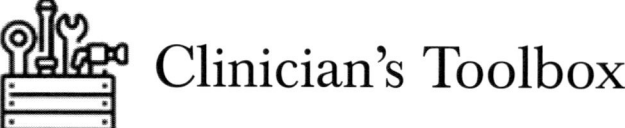

Clinician's Toolbox

- Family Bridges Website – www.buildingfaamilybridges.com.
- Turning Points for Families – https://lindagottlieb.com/.
- Kathleen Reay - Home (drkathleenreay.com).

Chapter 12

PROFESSIONAL LIABILITY AND PROTECTING YOURSELF

> **Learning Objectives:**
> 1. Understand the professional risks involved for MHP working with high-conflict divorce.
> 2. Understand the different formats for testifying.
> 3. Be able to identify how clinicians can violate licensing requirements.
> 4. Understand the importance of evaluating treatment effectiveness.
> 5. Know the guidelines for court-involved therapists.

Providing services to families going through divorce can involve interactions with a system that is much more adversarial than what mental health providers are used to. While many marriages dissolve somewhat reasonably with minimal conflict, others are highly litigious. The acrimony between the parents and lawyers can negatively affect clinicians working with the family.

Throughout this book, we have tried to describe the continuum of conflict possible within these families. When parents have minimal conflict during divorce and separation, they will likely seek counseling and support for their children together. Any mental health professional helping this family would probably feel comfortable interacting with both parents and would not need to have conversations with lawyers or worry about files being subpoenaed or being asked to testify. When parents are not communicating or doing so sporadically, counseling and support services may be recommended by an attorney or the court, or one parent may try to get counseling started without consulting the other parent. These are the types of situations that can create increased professional risks for clinicians.

The situations that entail the greatest risks involve custody litigation, where both parents ask for the primary custodial rights over the children. In these situations, one parent is likely to be disappointed at the end of the litigation and may have extreme reactions to the "loss" of parental time and control over the children. These parents can be so enraged that they blame the professionals in the case for their loss. Firm and clear professional boundaries, taking the time to read court orders, responding timely to legal correspondence, and being prepared to hire and/or consult with licensing boards and professional attorneys, will decrease potential liability.

Dr. Richard Warshak (2020) published a journal article describing the risks to professionals working with alienated children. He stated that the risks in working with this population may be related to working in an "emerging area of practice." The following risks were identified in his article: "false accusations of mistreating children; negatively biased commentary and sensationalists attacks in print, broadcasts, social media, professional conferences, journals, and in courtroom testimony; harassment, character assassination, and invasion of privacy; threats of violence and public humiliation; shunning and rumor spreading by colleagues and complaints to regulatory agencies" (p. 433).

These may seem extreme, but when one considers that the population of severely alienated children often includes psychologically compromised parents, it follows that professionals working with the family may also be affected by the parent's psychopathology. Remember from previous chapters, when a child rejects a parent completely for unjustified reasons, they have often been the victims of psychologically abusive parenting that can include threatening the child, implanting false memories, coaching, and other emotionally manipulative tactics (Bernet et al., 2016; Warshak, 2013; Warshak, 2020; Clawar & Rivlin, 2013). A parent who harms a child in this way to meet their own needs for control and/or revenge is severely disordered. Therefore, it should not be surprising that these parents would turn their rage onto the providers who opposed them in some way during the court process.

Social Media

Social media has increased the likelihood that parents displeased with a professional's work during the pendency of their case will air their grievances publicly. One way to deal with false information in an online review is to contact the review site and let them know that someone in a high-conflict custody battle posted the review and that the statements in the review are false. This may be enough for the site to remove the review. Another option is to ask the opposing party to write a review from their perspective, which will, at a minimum, provide another perspective of your work. It is not unusual in these cases that one parent leaves the courthouse extremely pleased with the outcome and all the professionals, while the other party leaves thinking the system and professionals are corrupt. Professionals working with this population may find that keeping online ratings at a three- or four-star level requires some effort and vigilance.

Mental health professionals can emotionally protect themselves from social media attacks by staying somewhat removed from them. Often, these reviews and posts include blatant lies and name-calling, which can cause a great deal of distress. One way to create some distance is to have an administrative assistant, office manager, or other staff member conduct periodic reviews of sites and social media posts directed at the provider. The same staff member can be responsible for getting the review removed or dealing with it in another way.

Continuing Education

The risks of working in an emerging area of practice can be mitigated by clinicians ensuring that they are keeping up with the new research on parental alienation and using approaches that have been cited in the work of scholars in the field. Forty percent of what we know about PA has been published since 2016 (Harman et al., 2022). Clinicians who have not been reading the literature on this topic recently may not have current information. While parental alienation has been established as a mature area of science, the empirical basis for treatment is not as robust. However, there are published journal articles on treatment of parent-child contact issues ranging in severity from mild to severe, and there are also books written by seasoned professionals about their clinical approach to this population (Polak, 2020; Baker et al. 2020;

Garber, 2021; Warshak, 2020; Judge & Deutsh, 2017; Friedlander & Walters, 2010; Greenberg et al., 2019; Smith, 2016).

Most of this book's treatment goals and techniques are based on peer-reviewed literature meant to increase clinicians' confidence in their treatment strategies and plans. The authors also know from experience that successfully defending treatment choices to regulatory boards or in cross-examination in court is much easier when treatment strategies are supported in scholarly publications. The citations in this book include publications through the year 2023. Clinicians can most easily stay abreast of new information by attending conferences and subscribing to journals that focus on working with divorcing families. Association of Families and Conciliation Courts (AFCC), the Parental Alienation Study Group (PASG), and The International Council on Shared Parenting (ICSP) are three associations that the authors have found to provide useful and current information.

Review Treatment Progress

Dr. Warshak's article (2020) on the risks and realities for professionals working with this population suggests that practitioners review the efficacy of their work regularly when working with parental alienation because the research has shown that traditional outpatient therapy is not effective with this population (Miller, 2013). He suggests that clinicians cease treatment if they do not see a decrease in the child's resistance to the parent within three months. In Dr. Kathleen Reay's article on The Family Reflections Reunification Program (2015), she provided a list of ten evidence-based reasons why traditional therapy does not work with a severe case of parental alienation:

1. Cases of parental alienation tend to be highly counterintuitive to anyone who is not a specialist or subspecialist in alienation and estrangement (Miller, 2013).
2. The treatment for severely alienated children and their family members is entirely different from that of mild or moderate alienation cases (Gardner et al., 2006).
3. Numerous therapists who are not trained in the specialized techniques that these families require often fall into the trap of believing the alienating parent and the programmed child and make the egregious mistake of contributing to the problem.

This phenomenon is often referred to as "third-party alienation" (Garber, 2004).

4. Some therapists will team up with the alienating parent and the alienated child. The target parent is excluded. In doing so, these clinicians run the risk of creating complete family annihilation. They get so caught up in the alienator and child's manipulation and delusional thinking that they lose sight of the realities of parental alienation. They may even form a strong bias against the target parent.
5. Untrained child protection workers and clinicians may not be able to accurately assess the differences between true allegations of child abuse and false allegations of child abuse that are commonly seen in severe cases of parental alienation (Sauber, 2010).
6. Parents who make false allegations of child abuse, conceivably those who are obsessively determined to annihilate the child's relationship with the target parent, are likely to demonstrate characteristics of various personality disorders – in particular, borderline personality disorder, narcissistic personality disorder, paranoid personality disorder, or sociopathic traits (Darnall, 2010; Gardner et al., 2006; Lorandos et al., 2013; Miller, 2013).
7. In severe cases, the alienating parent and alienated child are too determined and too delusional to respond to any form of traditional therapy (Fidler et al., 2013).
8. In court-ordered and non-court-ordered cases, alienating parents will fire therapists who question their motives and actions. If the therapy is focused on improving the relationship between the child and the rejected parent, then the favored parent will stop the child from seeking further interventions. It is not uncommon for alienating parents to "shop around" for clinicians who will eventually buy into their delusional thinking and manipulative games.
9. In court-ordered and non-court-ordered cases, alienating parents and alienated children are typically not motivated to attend therapy. They are obsessively determined to undermine both the therapist and the therapy (Darnall, 2010; Fidler et al., 2013; Miller, 2013; Reay, 2011; Sauber, 2010).
10. In traditional therapeutic settings, no attempt is made to physically remove the severely alienated child from the toxic home environment. The therapist attempts to influence the child

for one hour a week while the child continues to reside with the alienating parent for the rest of the week (Miller, 2013, p. 200).

Court-Ordered Therapy

The court order is the first document the clinician can use to set boundaries with parents because it should describe their professional role. It may also include directives to the parents, such as signing HIPAA releases for other professionals, requiring a certain number of sessions per week or month, and requiring the parents to follow the clinician's recommendations regarding treatment. When lawyers have agreed to appoint you in a therapeutic role and contacted you to ensure your interest and availability, you can ask that they include specific things in the court order defining your role and the clients' expectations. Some suggestions are:

- Naming who is responsible for your fees or how it should be divided between the parents.
- Requiring the parents to sign your paperwork and have it returned within a certain amount of time.
- Requirements to sign HIPAA releases for current and previous mental health professionals.
- Naming which family member(s) are expected to participate in the therapy.
- Stating whether both parents should share in bringing the child to therapy.
- Stating whether the child can miss school for therapeutic appointments.

There are two kinds of court orders: temporary orders and final orders. Temporary orders are just what the name implies. They are meant to be in place only for a while. They are intended to apply to the current family situation. Sometimes, a temporary order remains in place for several years, but this is not the norm.

A final order represents the parties' final agreements or the court's final ruling and contains the rules that the family abides by unless the parents mutually agree to do something different or a parent files a motion to modify the order. When a parent files for a modification, the rules in the final order remain in place until the court hears the facts for the request to modify or until the parties agree to change the previous order.

Provisions for counseling can be included in temporary and final orders. Clinicians should always ask for the *current* order from parents. It is common in protracted divorce situations for several versions of a temporary order to be issued before the final order is issued. Clinicians should ensure that they have the most recent court order and that the judge signs it.

The most important sections to review are parenting time schedules (also called possession and access), decision-making rights, parenting duties, and any special provisions described for counseling and other mental health services, which are generally contained in a separate paragraph in the order under a subheading such as "*Provisions for therapy*" Mutual decision-making rights require the parents to agree before continuing with services. Exclusive or sole decision-making rights give one parent the right to decide on the issue, with or without the other parent's agreement. Sometimes, sole decision-making rights require that the parent "confer" with the other parent before making the decision. When it comes to psychological and psychiatric care, clinicians must ensure that the parent setting up services for the child abides by the order. Otherwise, the counselor could be held responsible for seeing the child without the appropriate parental authority. In Texas, these provisions are contained within a section entitled "*Rights and Duties.*" Clinicians should become familiar with the format and subheadings of the separation and divorce orders in their state.

It is common for highly contested divorce cases to include specific parameters for mental health professionals. The specificity related to mental health services can vary from something as general as stating that the child should be in individual therapy to something as specific as naming the professional to provide the services, defining a start date and requiring a certain number of sessions per week or per month, and defining how the parents should share the costs.

The Association of Families and Conciliation Courts (AFCC) has provided the following definitions for court-involved therapy (AFCC, 2010):

- Court-Involved Therapist (CIT): Any mental health professional providing psychotherapeutic treatment of a parent, child, couple

or family who is, at any time during the treatment, involved with the legal system.
- Court-Appointed Therapist: Any mental health professional providing psychotherapeutic treatment of a parent, child, couple or family undertaken because the particular psychotherapist was ordered by a judge to provide treatment. The Court order designates the specific psychotherapist and may describe the expected treatment.
- Court-Ordered Therapist: Any mental health professional providing psychotherapeutic treatment of a parent, child, couple or family undertaken because it was ordered by a judge. The Court order does not designate a specific therapist and may describe the expected treatment (p. 2).

Other aspects of mental health services that may also be addressed in the order are whether the parents are required to follow recommendations made by the MHP, therapeutic goals, and parental access to the records, among other things. The AFCC 2010 guidelines for court-involved therapy recommend that clinicians understand the extent to which the court expects them to be involved. The only way that a clinician will know this is to review the court order thoroughly. Consultations with the lawyers and/or the guardian ad litem or the child's attorney are also recommended as a process by which clinicians can better understand what is being asked of them in any particular case.

It may seem strange that a court order would outline therapeutic goals. Still, when other professionals like guardian ad litems, co-parenting counseling, parenting facilitators, lawyers, and mediators are trying to get parents to cooperate and share time with their children, they may define some of the therapeutic goals to ensure that parents understand that the purpose of therapy is to create positive relationships between both parents and the kids and to get the kids on parenting time schedules that include time at both parents' homes. When one parent has used therapy for the children as a way to further a narrative that the other parent should have limited time or stall the progression of the divorce, the attorneys may craft precise orders so that the parent understands the primary goal of therapy is for the kids to move consistently between two homes. The authors have found this more helpful than intrusive, particularly when dealing with parents who attempt to bias or pressure the clinician to support limiting contact between the child and the other parent or who use their own therapy to re-hash an outdated or false narrative about the other parent.

Professional Role Boundaries

When we are training other mental health professionals to do this work, they emphasize the importance of "staying in your lane." This is very important in terms of professional protection and adhering to the court order. In high-conflict cases, multiple professionals are often appointed or hired to work with a family – individual therapists for children and/or parents, co-parenting therapists, parenting coaches, psychological evaluators, guardian ad litems, and family therapists. The second guideline in the AFCC (2010) guidelines emphasizes the importance for counselors to maintain boundaries according to their role. One of the mistakes we see happen most often is counseling professionals working with children getting pressured into making statements about custody and parenting time schedules. Clinicians cannot make parenting time and custody recommendations without conducting a custody evaluation. Regardless of your thoughts on the matter or how long you have been working with the child, doing so would be "stepping out of your lane." Therefore, if a lawyer asks you if the child should stop seeing one of the parents or increase their time with one of the parents, you should decline to answer, stating something like, "It is outside the scope of my work to answer that question." Stating an opinion on this type of question could be a quick way to receive a board complaint.

Lawyers will often want to make the child's therapist or the reunification therapist the arbiter of the child's time spent with the parent they are resisting. While this may make sense to all the parties during final negotiations, it compromises the clinician's relationship with the child and their licensing requirements. Therapists can recommend to lawyers that they keep a guardian ad litem or the child's attorney in place to continue to make parenting time recommendations as the child's relationship with the parent improves.

Professionals providing individual services to children should stay attuned to requests from lawyers and parents who would morph their roles into those of family therapists. As outlined in other chapters, it is at times necessary and appropriate for a child's therapist to have a joint session between the child and a parent; however, when this happens too frequently, it could be asserted by a disgruntled lawyer or parent that the clinician is playing a dual role – that of individual therapist and family therapist. If the parent and the child need regular and ongoing joint sessions, the clinician should make a referral for family therapy.

Providing services to one parent and the child when the clinician's appointed role is as the child's therapist can also interfere with the clinician's rapport and trust with the other parent. The child's clinician should strive to balance and equalize their contact with each parent. Neutrality, in this regard, is extremely important.

Assessing Treatment Effectiveness

Warshak (2020) identified risks to clinicians working with children who are aligned with one parent and rejecting another. He recommended that clinicians working with this population ensure that their knowledge of treatment options includes an understanding of what type of treatment is appropriate for different levels of rejection (discussed as mild, moderate, and severe in the preceding treatment chapters); understand and be able to explain the limitations, benefits, and risks associated with the type of intervention being offered (i.e., informed consent); and know when to terminate. Rejected parents who see a clinician as continuing to provide services that are not resulting in an improved relationship with their children or increased willingness for the child to spend more time with them may see the clinician as prolonging the trauma to the child and be inclined to file a complaint.

Providing effective treatment for this population requires specialized training. AFCC (2010) guideline 3.2 discusses the need for clinicians working in court-involved therapy to have knowledge in the following areas:

1. Characteristics of divorcing/separated families and children (2) Family systems and other systems in which court-involved families interact (3) The impact of high interparental conflict on post-separation custody arrangements (4) Effective interventions with divorcing or separated families (5) Adaptations of traditional therapeutic approaches that may be necessary to work with divorcing or separated families (6) Characteristics and needs of special populations who may be involved in treatment (7) Ethical issues and applicable local legal standards (pp. 9-10).

Graduate school training may suffice for the first two knowledge areas but will not prepare clinicians for the other five areas.

Clinicians should consider regularly evaluating their attempts to improve the relationship between a parent and a child, document improvements, or lack thereof, and refer the family for a higher level of care or additional services when there is little to no documentation of improvements. Consultations with colleagues are also recommended when evaluating the need for continued therapy when a lack of progress is a concern. AFCC (2010) guideline 8.8 states that clinicians should obtain advice, "When in doubt about an appropriate course of action, the CIT should consider seeking legal advice or professional consultation. Such advice may protect the clients in therapy and the CIT" (p. 25).

Testifying in Court

If the family is scheduled to go to court and the clinician is going to provide testimony, the lawyer requesting the clinician's testimony should issue a subpoena. This is another way the clinician can maintain a neutral stance between the parents and their lawyers. If an attorney calls the professional to check their availability for court, the professional should request that the attorney issue a subpoena for their appearance. Subpoenas cost money and lawyers will try to save on the expense to their client by merely calling the professional or requesting to serve the subpoena by email. The best way to maintain neutrality is to request that the subpoena be served to the professional by a process server. When time is of the essence, a subpoena issued by email is fine.

Professionals should read the subpoena thoroughly for time, place, and other requirements. A subpoena may be requesting records delivered to an attorney's office by a specific date and time. It may request your presence at a court hearing or the professional's presence at the hearing and require the professional to bring their records. If the professional cannot abide by the request, they are required to notify the lawyer issuing the subpoena. If a clinician believes that releasing the record would place their client in emotional harm or violate private health care information, they are required to notify the lawyer.

It is important for clinicians working with this population to identify a lawyer they can use when faced with legal requests for documents and/or court appearances that they believe would harm their clients.

Clinicians usually have coverage for legal services included in their professional liability coverage. You should know the annual limits on these services and be willing to obtain legal advice from lawyers specializing in the professional liability of mental health providers. When dealing with a particularly aggressive lawyer who seems intent on damaging your credibility, you should consult with your professional liability attorney regarding all written and verbal communication. Disgruntled attorneys often represent disgruntled clients who are also looking for areas where the clinician has erred so they can file board complaints. If your attorney oversees your communications, they can protect you if the parent files a complaint.

It has been our experience that there are usually a small number of MHPs doing this work in metropolitan areas around the country; therefore, any clinician interested in pursuing work with this population should inquire about the other professionals in the area specializing in families going through separation and divorce. The support from those other providers will be extremely beneficial. They will know the name(s) of the professional liability lawyers in the area, the family law attorneys who are easiest to work with, and provide a newer MHP with referrals to help build a clientele. They are also a source of guidance, providing feedback and assurance that the newer MHP's course of treatment is appropriate. New graduates considering this kind of work should consider a supervisor who has experience providing mental health services within the context of family law.

Interfacing with the legal system can feel intimidating. It is expected to be nervous about receiving a subpoena, being deposed, and being asked to provide testimony at a hearing. Do not expect that these things will come easy or feel comfortable right away. Providing testimony and communicating with lawyers are activities that will require practice, time, and patience. Some MHPs go to court one time and decide they do not ever want to do it again. In contrast, others will be curious about the process, see it as a challenge, and/or view their testimony as a critical piece of information and thus worth the stress to help the child and family.

There are different forms of "sworn testimony" that can be provided by MHPs. Affidavits are written statements signed by a notary. A deposition provides oral testimony, usually given in a lawyer's office. A court hearing provides for testimony to be delivered orally in a courtroom. Do not ever underestimate the value of your insight and work with the client in the court proceedings. While there may be one attorney who does not want to know what the MHP has to offer, we have found that most judges appreciate the information provided by clinicians and consider it when making decisions for the family. One exception to this is when clinicians allow themselves to become advocates for one parent's position rather than providing factual information to the court about their clinical work with the family. Judges typically give more credibility to witnesses that present information in a balanced and neutral way.

A lawyer may ask the MHP to write an affidavit describing concerns and the extent of their treatment of the client. An affidavit can be used to replace oral testimony when the attorney is faced with an emergency situation threatening the safety of the client and there is no time to schedule a hearing. The attorney may be requesting immediate intervention from the court. The MHP's affidavit would likely contain facts based on their treatment of the client or concerns about the health and safety of the client. The intervention requested could be to restrict contact between a child and one of their parents, to restrict contact between parents, or some higher level of care for the client. Clinicians should guard against any statement recommending a restriction of access between a child and a parent. The affidavit may offer facts obtained in therapy or even concern about the child's welfare but should not go as far as recommending that the child not have contact or have less contact. The decision about parental access is one for the judge to make based on the facts presented to the judge. The attorney must make the case that the child is in threat of immediate danger in the care of a parent. The MHP's affidavit may contain some of the facts used to make that case but should not contain recommendations about possession and access.

There are other court-appointed roles that allow for custody and possession (or parenting time) recommendations. States may refer to these roles with different titles but in general they are usually non-therapeutic roles such as attorney ad litem, guardian ad litem, custody evaluator, or parenting coordinator. When a professional has one of these titles, the MHP can discuss their concerns with the professional, who can then make recommendations to the lawyers and/or the court.

An affidavit could also be requested when the MHP will not be available on the day of the hearing to provide oral testimony, but the attorney believes that the knowledge the MHP has about their client is important to share with the court. Attorneys may offer to draft the affidavit based on their knowledge of the MHP's opinions and observations. This is fine as long as the attorney forwards the affidavit to the MHP for review and editing. Affidavits need to be in a particular format so the lawyer's offer to get it started probably saves them time in the long run. The clinician should correct false and exaggerated statements and not allow an attorney to overly skew their opinion to try and make their case.

Providing testimony in a deposition can feel slightly less intimidating than going to court. A deposition can be conducted with a MHP virtually or in person. The question-and-answer format is less rigid than being in court, and the venue is usually more relaxed. The answers provided can be more explanatory and do not necessarily need to adhere to a "yes or no" format, although there may be benefits to keeping the answers brief. The attorney's questions also do not need to be as succinct as they may be in a trial. In the authors' experience, attorneys sometimes use a deposition as a "fishing expedition" to find out everything the clinician may know about. This decreases the likelihood that the attorney will be surprised by information provided by the MHP in court and allows them to better prepare their cross-examination questions for the MHP. The questions may be things the MHP does not know about, and when this is the case, "I do not know" is a perfectly acceptable answer. Another acceptable answer is, "I need to think about that." If the MHP cannot remember, it is acceptable to say, "I can't remember, but I am happy to look at my notes and get back to you with the answer." A deposition can also be helpful to the clinician as it gives you an idea of what kinds of questions to expect if you eventually have to testify in court.

Despite the more relaxed environment, we recommend that clinicians remain aware that a court reporter records their answers and can be used during a court hearing. A deposed witness can and should request a copy of their deposition transcript for review. This request can be made at the deposition. Sometimes, the court reporter will ask if the witness would like a copy of the transcript. If there are mistakes in the testimony, either factual errors or transcription errors, the witness can submit a request for their answers to be corrected. If the answers provided in court testimony differ from those provided in the deposition, the attorney will bring that out in court, and it can hurt the witness' credibility when there is not a logical explanation for the change in the testimony.

The subpoena requesting the deposition should state whether it will be virtual or in person and provide an address when the deposition is in person. In most cases, the clinician knows a lawyer is trying to depose them because the lawyer has tried to ascertain their availability. If the lawyer has scheduled the deposition without consulting with you, it is perfectly acceptable to notify the lawyer that you are unavailable and offer other dates.

Clinicians should calculate the time they will spend preparing, traveling, and being deposed and ask the client to pay them for that time before the deposition occurs. It can be difficult to collect payment after the deposition or the court hearing, regardless of the outcome. This can seem unusual to clinical providers used to collecting payment after services. Attorneys usually require clients to have funds for hearings in their account before trying the case. The authors recommend that clinicians do the same for fees related to providing testimony.

Whether the MHP is preparing to give testimony in a deposition or in a court hearing, they should take the time to review their case file thoroughly. Some lawyers ensure that all their witnesses are prepared and know what to expect in the form of questions they will be asked on the stand. Clinicians appreciate this, especially when their case file is relatively large because it is easier to prepare and commit to memory facts and examples that are valuable for the court to know. In most hearings, the witness does not bring a case file up to the stand. The information they offer is usually committed to memory. The lawyer may help refresh your memory by offering emails, case notes, or other correspondence to review during your testimony. Clinicians should always know their treatment start date, their last session date, and how many sessions they have had with each family member. As stated previously, it is acceptable to say you do not remember or do not know the answer to a question. It is also acceptable to offer to look at your notes during a break and provide the answer when you return to court.

Clinicians usually serve as fact witnesses. A fact witness has firsthand knowledge about the case. Clinicians testify to the facts they know through observations and interactions with the people involved in the case. They do not usually offer opinions unless they have been qualified as an expert. An expert witness is someone who may or may not have reviewed the facts related to the case. They have specialized knowledge about some aspects of the case. In family law matters experts are usually offering opinions on parenting plans, high-conflict dynamics that could be affecting the children, parental alienation, domestic violence, developmental needs of children, special needs of children, and custody, among other things.

The authors recommend that clinicians who are just beginning their work with divorcing families and not familiar with providing testimony, make efforts to consult with other mental health professionals who have some experience. Basic tips for providing testimony usually consist of listening closely to the question, only answering the question asked and not providing other information, and answering with yes or no whenever possible, especially when being cross-examined. The lawyer will ask you to explain your answer more in-depth or provide examples if they need the clinician to go beyond a yes or no answer. When you cannot answer with yes or no, it is acceptable to state that a yes or no answer is not possible. A simple rule of thumb to help you remember this is, "Answer the question asked." The lawyer will either ask you to explain, rephrase their question, or move on to another question.

A common strategy used in cross-examination to minimize the impact of testimony when the testimony does not support the lawyer's legal position is to ask the clinician hypothetical questions or possibility questions. The latter might sound like, "Isn't it possible that Suzie did not want her mother to join her therapy session because she is afraid of her mother?" If the clinician were to say no, that was not a possibility, the lawyer could come back with accusations of the clinician claiming they know more than they possibly could because how could they know *absolutely* that there was nothing else going on for the child? One way to answer this is to say, "It is possible but not probable based on what I know about the client." The authors also want to caution clinicians again to be watchful for attorneys asking custody and/or parenting time questions. Even questions that ask the clinician about their recommendations regarding phone access or phone schedules can be considered parenting time recommendations. The standard response from the clinical provider should be that they cannot answer questions about parenting time because it is outside the scope of their role.

In closing, clinical work that involves legal activity is not for everyone. Many clinicians do not accept families going through divorce as clients because of their hesitancy to be involved in litigation or work closely with lawyers. However, there are many points on the continuum of providing services within the family law context that do not require frequent testimony or interfacing with lawyers. An entire caseload does not need to be composed of families involved in litigation. However, there is an immense need for specialized providers in this area, and one's practice could quickly fill up with that population. It is also incredibly useful for these families to have support during this time. If clinicians were willing to dedicate even a small portion of their caseloads to serve these families, the differences they could make in the long-term outcomes for these parents and children could be immense.

 Clinician's Toolbox

- ✗ AFCC Guidelines for Court-Involved Therapy (GUIDELINES FOR COURT-INVOLVED THERAPY (afccnet.org).
- ✗ *Coping with Cross-Examination and other Pathways to Effective Testimony* by Stanley L. Brodsky.
- ✗ *The Expert Expert Witness: More Maxims and Guidelines for Testifying in Court* by Stanley L. Brodsky.

REFERENCES

Abidin, R. (1995). *Parenting Stress Index.* Psychological Assessment Resources Inc.

Abramowicz, S. (1999). Note: English child custody law, 1660-1839: The origins of judicial intervention in parental custody. *Columbia Law Review, 99*, 1334-1392. http://digitalcommons.wayne.edu/lawfrp/37

AFCC Task Force. (2011). Guidelines for court-involved therapy. *Family Court Review, 49*(3), 564-581.

Albertson-Kelly, J., & Burkhard, B. (2013). Family reunification in a forensic setting. In A. J. L. Baker & S. R. Sauber (Eds.), *Working with alienated children and families: A clinical guidebook* (pp. 232–251). Routledge.

Allen, S. (February 12, 2023). *Integrating parent coaching to enhance support in high conflict divorce.* [Training Presentation]. Allen & Associates.

American Psychiatric Association. (2013). *Diagnostic and statistical manual of mental disorders* (5th ed.). Washington, DC: Author. https://doi.org/10.1176/appi.books.9780890425596

American Psychological Association. (1996). *Violence and the Family. Report of the APA Presidential Task Force on Violence and the Family.* Washington, DC, USA: American Psychological Association.

Articles in peer-reviewed journals and published books on the Parental Alienation Syndrome (PAS), Richard A. Gardner, M. D. (2023). Richard Gardner. Retrieved on August 20, 2024, from https://richardagardner.com/pas_peerreviewarticles

Association of Family and Conciliation Courts (AFCC), Task Force on Court-Involved Therapy. (2011). Guidelines for court-involved therapy. *Family Court Review, 49*, 564-581.

Austin, W. G., & Drozd, L. M. (2013). Judge's bench book for application of the integrated framework for the assessment of intimate partner violence in child custody disputes. *Journal of Child Custody: Research, Issues, and Practices, 10*(2), 99-119. https://doi.org/10.1080/15379418.2013.796850

Baker, A. J. L. (2005). The long-term effects of parental alienation on adult children: A qualitative research study. *The American Journal of Family Therapy, 33*, 289-302. https://doi.org/10.1080/01926180590962129

Baker, A. J. L. (2007). *Adult children of parental alienation syndrome: Breaking the ties that Bind.* W.W. Norton & Co.

Baker, A. J. L. (2008). Even when you win you lose: Targeted parents' perceptions of their attorneys. *American Journal of Family Therapy, 38*(4), 292–309. https://doi.org/10.1080/01926187.2010.493429

Baker, A. J. L. (2010). Adult recall of parental alienation in a community sample: Prevalence and associations with psychological maltreatment. *Journal of Divorce & Remarriage, 51,* 16-35. https://doi.org/10.1080/10502550903423206

Baker, A. J. L. (2020). Parental alienation and empirical research. In D. Lorandos & W. Bernet (Eds.), *Parental alienation: Science and law* (pp. 207–253). Charles C Thomas Publisher, Ltd.

Baker, A. J. L. (2020). Reliability and validity of the four-factor model of parental alienation. *Journal of Family Therapy, 42*(1), 110–118. https://doi.org/10.1111/1467-6427.12253

Baker, A. J. L., & Andre, K. (2015). *Getting Through My Parents' Divorce: A Workbook for Children Coping with Divorce, Parental Alienation, and Loyalty Conflicts.* New Harbinger Publications.

Baker, A. J. L., & Ben-Ami, N. (2011). To turn a child against a parent is to turn a child against himself: The direct and indirect effects of exposure to parental alienation strategies on self-esteem and well-being. *Journal of Divorce & Remarriage, 52*(7), 472–489. https://doi.org/10.1080/10502556.2011.609424

Baker, A. J. L., Burkhard, B., & Albertson-Kelly, J. (2012). Differentiating alienated from not alienated children: A pilot study. *Journal of Divorce & Remarriage, 53*(3), 178–193. https://doi.org/10.1080/10502556.2012.663266

Baker, A. J. L., & Chambers, J. (2011). Adult recall of childhood exposure to parental conflict: Unpacking the black box of parental alienation. *Journal of Divorce & Remarriage, 52* (1), 55–76. https://doi.org/10.1080/10502556.2011.534396

Baker, A. J. L., & Darnall, D. C. (2006). Behaviors and strategies employed in parental alienation: A survey of parental experiences. *Journal of Divorce & Remarriage, 45*(1-2), 97–124. https://doi.org/10.1300/J087v45n01_06

Baker, A. J. L., & Darnall, D. C. (2007). A construct study of the eight symptoms of severe parental alienation syndrome: A survey of parental experiences. *Journal of Divorce & Remarriage, (47)*1/2, 55-75. Doi: 10.1300/J087v47n01_04

Baker, A. J. L., & Eichler, A. (2016). The linkage between parental alienation behaviors and child alienation. *Journal of Divorce & Remarriage, 57*(7), 475-484. https://doi.org/10.1080/10502556.2016.1220285

Baker, A. J. L., & Fine, P. R. (2008). *Beyond the high road: Responding to 17 parental alienation strategies without compromising your morals or harming your child.* Self Published eBook.

Baker, A. J. L., Miller, S., Bernet, W., & Adebayo, T. (2019). The assessment of attitudes and behaviors about physically abused children: A survey of mental health professionals. *Journal of Child and Family Studies, 28,* 3401-3401. https://10.1007/s10826-019-01522-5

Baker, A. J. L., Murray, C., & Adkins, K. (2020) Parameters of reunification therapy and predictors of treatment success in high conflict divorce cases: A survey of mental health professionals, *Journal of Divorce & Remarriage, 61*(8), 593-614. https://doi.org/10.1080/10502556.2020.1824206

Baker, A. J. L., & Schneiderman, M. (2015). *Bonded to the abuser: How victims make sense of childhood abuse*. Rowman & Littlefield.

Baker, A. J. L. & Verrocchio, M. C. (2014). Parental bonding and parental alienation as correlates of psychological maltreatment in adults in intact and non-intact families. *Journal of Child and Family Studies 24*(10), 3047-3057. Doi: 10.1007/s10826-014-0108-0

Baker, K., & Eichler, A. (2023). Child protection assessments. In D. Lorandos (Ed.), *Litigator's Handbook on Forensic Medicine, Psychiatry and Psychology*. West Group.

Bala, N. M. C., Mitnick, M., Trocmé, N., & Houston, C. (2007). Sexual abuse allegations and parental separation: Smokescreen or fire? *Journal of Family Studies, 13*(1), 26-56. https://doi.org/10.5172/jfs.327.13.1.26

Baude, A., Pearson, J., & Drapeau, S. (2016). Child adjustment in joint physical custody versus sole custody: A meta-analytic review. *Journal of Divorce and Remarriage, 57*(5), 338-360.

Beach, S. R. H., & Whisman, M. A. (2013) Relationship distress: Impact on mental illness, physical health, children, and family economics. In: H. M. Foran, S. R. H. Beach, A. M. S. Slep, R. E. Heyman, & M. Z. Wambolt, (Eds.), *Family Problems and Family Violence: Reliable Assessment and the ICD-11* (pp. 91-100). Springer Publishing.

Beck, A. T., Epstein, N., Brown, G., & Steer, R. A. (1988). An inventory for measuring clinical anxiety: psychometric properties. *Journal of Consulting and Clinical Psychology, 56,* 893–897. [PubMed: 3204199]

Beck, Steer, & Brown, (1996). Beck depression inventory (BDI–II). Second ed. Psychological Corporation.

Ben-Ami, N. & Baker, A. J. L. (2012). The long-term correlates of childhood exposure to parental alienation on adult self-sufficiency and well-being. *American Journal of Family Therapy, 40,* 169-183. https://doi.org/10.1080/01926187.2011.601206

Benedek, E. P., & Schetky, D. H. (1985). Custody and visitation: Problems and perspectives. *The Psychiatric Clinics of North America, 8*(4), 857-873.

Bernet W. & Greenhill, L. L. (2022). The Five-Factor model for the diagnosis of parental alienation. *Journal of the American Academy of Child and Adolescent Psychiatry 61*(5), 591–594. https://doi.org/10.1016/j.jaac.2021.11.026

Bernet, W. (2006). Sexual abuse allegations in the context of child custody disputes. In R.A. Gardner, S.R. Sauber, and D. Lorandos (Eds.). *The International Handbook of Parental Alienation Syndrome: Conceptual, Legal, and Clinical Considerations* (pp. 242-263). Charles C. Thomas, Publisher, Ltd.

Bernet, W., Baker, A. J. L., & Adkins, K. L. (2022) Definitions and terminology regarding child alignments, estrangement, and alienation: A survey of custody evaluators. *Journal of Forensic Sciences, 67*(1), 279-288. https://doi.org/10.1111/1556-4029.14868

Bernet, W., Gregory, N., Reay, K. M., & Rohner, R. P. (2018). An objective measure of splitting in parental alienation: the parental acceptance–rejection questionnaire. *Journal of Forensic Sciences, 63*(3), 776–783. https://doi.org/10.1111/1556-4029.13625

Bernet, W., Gregory, N., Rohner, R. P., & Reay, K. M. (2020). Measuring the difference between parental alienation and parental estrangement: The PARQ-Gap. *Journal of Forensic Sciences, 65*(4), 1225–1234. https://doi.org/10.1111/1556-4029.14300

Bernet, W., Wamboldt, M. Z., Narrow, W. E. (2016). Child affected by parental relationship distress. *Journal of the American Academy of Child and Adolescent Psychiatry, 55*(7). https://doi.org/10.1016/j.jaac.2016.04.018

Blagg, N., & Godfrey, E. (2018). Exploring parent-child relationships in alienated versus neglected/emotionally abused children using the Bene-Anthony Family Relations Test. *Child Abuse Review, 27*(6), 486–496. https://doi.org/10.1002/car.2537

Boss, P. (1999). *Ambiguous loss: Learning to live with unresolved grief.* Harvard University Press.

Boss, P. (2006). *Loss, trauma, and resilience: Therapeutic work with ambiguous loss.* W.W. Norton & Company.

Boss, P. (2022). *The myth of closure: Ambiguous loss in a time of pandemic and change.* W.W. Norton & Company.

Boss, P., Bryant, C. M., & Mancini, J. A. (2017). *Family stress management: A contextual approach* (3rd ed.). Sage Publications.

Bowen, M. (1961). The family as the unit of study and treatment: Workshop, 1959: 1. Family psychotherapy. *American Journal of Orthopsychiatry, 31*(1), 40 – 60. https://doi.org/10.1111/j.1939-0025.1961.tb02106.x

Bowlby, J. (1969). *Attachment.* Basic Books.

Bowlby, J. (1988). *A secure base: Parent-child attachment and healthy human development.* Basic Books.

Brown, T. (2003). Fathers and child abuse allegations in the context of parental separation and divorce. *Family Court Review, 41*(3), 367-380. https://doi.org/10.1111/j.174-1617.2003.tb00898.x

Bruck, M. & Ceci, S. J. (1995). Amicus brief for the case of State of New Jersey v. Michaels presented by Committee of Concerned Social Scientists. *Psychology, Public Policy, and Law, 1*(2), 272–322. https://doi.org/10.1037/1076-8971.1.2.272

Cartwright, G. (2006). Beyond parental alienation syndrome: Reconciling the alienated child and the lost parent. In R. Gardner, R. Sauber, and D. Lorandos (Eds.), *The International Handbook of Parental Alienation Syndrome* (pp. 286-290). Charles C. Thomas, Publisher, Ltd.

Ceci, S. J., & Bruck, M. (1993). Suggestibility of the child witness: A historical review and synthesis. *Psychological Bulletin, 113*(3), 403–439. https://doi.org/10.1037/0033-2909.113.3.403

Ceci, S. J., & Bruck, M. (1995). Jeopardy in the courtroom: A scientific analysis of children's testimony. American Psychological Association.

Chapman, G.D. (2010). *The five love languages,* Walker Large Print.

Chapsky v. Wood, 26 Kan. 650 (1881). Chapsky v. Wood - Kansas - Case Law – VLEX 901133222

Children rights. Travis County, Texas. (n.d.). https://www.traviscountytx.gov/dro/children-rights

Clawar, S. S., & Rivlin, B. V. (2013). Children held hostage: Identifying brainwashed children, presenting a case, and crafting solutions. American Bar Association.

Commonwealth v. Addicks, 5 Binney 520 (1813). Commonwealth v. Addicks - Pennsylvania - Case Law - VLEX 900299706

Cyr, C., Euser, E.M., Bakersmans-Kranenburg, M. J., & Van Ijzendoorn, M. H. (2010). Attachment security and disorganization in maltreating and high-risk families: A series of meta-analyses. *Development & Psychopathology 22*(1), 87-108. https://doi.org/10.1017/S0954579409990289

Dattilio, F. M., & Nichols, M. P. (2011). Reuniting estranged family members: A cognitive-behavioral-systemic perspective. *American Journal of Family Therapy, 39*(2), 88–99. https://doi.org/10.1080/01926187.2010.530169

De Bono, Edward. (1999). *Six thinking hats* (Revised and Updated). Back Bay Books.

de Manneville v. de Manneville, 32 Eng. Rep. 762 (1804). De Manneville v De Manneville. [HIGH COURT of CHANCERY] - Case Law - VLEX 805405485

Demby, S. (2009). Interparent hatred and its impact on parenting: Assessment in forensic custody evaluations. *Psychoanalytic Inquiry, 29*(6), 477–490. https://doi.org/10.1080/07351690903013959

Despert, J. L. (1953). *Children of Divorce*. The Country Life Press.

Drozd, L., Olesen, N., & Saini, M. A. (2013). *Parenting plan & child custody evaluations: Using decision trees to increase evaluator competence & avoid preventable errors*. Professional Resource Press.

Dunne, J. & Hedrick, M. (1994). The parental alienation syndrome: An analysis of sixteen selected cases. *Journal of Divorce & Remarriage, 21*(3/4), 21-38.

Eddy, W. A., Burns, A., & Chafin, K. (2020). *Biff for coparent communication: Your guide to difficult texts, emails, and social media posts*. Unhooked Books, an imprint of High Conflict Institute Press.

El Sheikh, M., Cummings, E. M., Kouros, C. D., Elmore-Staton, L., & Buckhalt, J. (2008). Marital psychological and physical aggression and children's mental and physical health: Direct, mediated, and moderated effects. *Journal of Consulting & Clinical Psychology, 76*(1), 138–148. https://doi-org.dewey.umhb.edu/10.1037/0022-006X.76.1.138

Festinger, L. (1957). *A theory of cognitive dissonance*. Stanford University Press.

Fidler, B. J., & Bala, N. (2010). Children resisting post-separation contact with a parent: concepts, controversies and conundrums. *Family Court Review, 48*(1), 10–47. https://doi.org/10.1111/j.1744-1617.2009.01287.x

Fidler, B.J. & Bala, N. (2020). Concepts, controversies and conundrums of "Alienation": Lessons learned in a decade and reflections on challenges ahead. *Family Court Review, 58*, 576-603. https://doi.org/10.1111/fcre.12488

Fidler, B. J., & Ward, P. (2016). Clinical decision-making in parent-child contact problem cases: Tailoring the intervention to the family's needs. In A. M. Judge & R. M. Deutsch (Eds.), *Overcoming parent-child contact problems: Family-based interventions for resistance, rejection and alienation* (pp. 13–62). Oxford University Press.

Fidler, B. J., Bala, N., & Saini, M. A. (2013). *Children who resist post-separation parental contact: A differential approach for legal and mental health professionals.* American psychology-law society series. Oxford University Press.

Fidler, B. J., Deutch, R., & Polak, S. (2019). "How am I supposed to treat these cases?" Working with families struggling with entrenched parent-child contact problems: A hybrid case. In L. R. Greenberg, B. J. Fidler, & M. A. Saini (Eds.), *Evidence-informed interventions for court-involved families: Promoting healthy coping and development,* (pp. 227-259). Oxford University Press.

Fidnick, L. S., & Deutsch, R. M. (2012). An introduction to the AFCC guidelines for court-involved therapy. *Journal of Child Custody, 9*(1–2), 5–10. https://doi.org/10.1080/15379418.2012.652564

Fraiberg, S., Adelson, E., Shapiro, V. (1975). Ghosts in the nursery. A psychoanalytic approach to the problems of impaired infant-mother relationships. *Journal of American Academy of Child Psychiatry, 14*(3), 387-421. https://doi.org/10.1016/s0002-7138(09)61442-4

Frankl, V. (1963). *Man's search for meaning.* Beacon Press.

Freeman, B. W. (2020). The psychosocial assessment of contact refusal. In D. Lorandos, and W. Bernet (Eds.), *Parental alienation: Science and law* (pp. 44-81). Charles C. Thomas, Publisher, Ltd.

Freeman, R., Abel, D., Cowper-Smith, M., & Stein, L. (2004). Reconnecting children with absent parents: A model for intervention. *Family Court Review, 42,* 439–459.

Freud, S. (1917). *A difficulty in the path of psychoanalysis. Collected works* (vol. 17). Hogarth.

Friedlander, S. and Walters, M.G. (2010), When a child rejects a parent: Tailoring the intervention to fit the problem. *Family Court Review, 48,* 98-111. https://doi.org/10.1111/j.1744-1617.2009.01291.x

Garber B. D. & Simon, R. A. (2023). Looking beyond the sorting hat: Deconstructing the "Five Factor Model" of parental alienation. *Family Transitions, 65*(1), 5-31. https://doi.org/10.1080/10502556.2023.2262359

Garber, B. D. (2011). Parental alienation and the dynamics of the enmeshed parent-child dyad: Adultification, parentification, and infantilization. *Family Court Review, 49,* 322–335.

Garber, B. D. (2015). Cognitive-behavioral methods in high-conflict divorce: Systematic desensitization adapted to parent-child reunification interventions. *Family Court Review, 53,* 96 –112. http://dx.doi.org/10.1111/fcre.12133

Garber, B. D. (2021). *Mending Fences: A collaborative cognitive-behavioral reunification protocol serving the best interests of the post-divorce, polarized child.* Unhooked Books.

Gardner, R. A. (1985). Recent trends in divorce and custody litigation. *The Academy Forum, 29*(2), 3-7.

Gardner, R. A. (1992). *The parental alienation syndrome: A guide for mental health and legal professionals.* (1st ed.). Creative Therapeutics, Inc.

Gardner, R. A. (1998). Recommendations for dealing with parents who induce a parental alienation syndrome in their children. *Journal of Divorce & Remarriage, 28*(3-4), 1–23. https://doi.org/10.1300/J087v28n03_01

Gardner, R. A. (1998). *The parental alienation syndrome: A guide for mental health and legal professionals* (2nd ed.). Creative Therapeutics, Inc.

Gardner, R. A. (2001). Should courts order PAS children to visit/reside with the alienated parent? A follow-up study. *American Journal of Forensic Psychology, 19*(3), 61–106.

Gardner, R. A. (2002). Parental alienation syndrome vs. parental alienation: Which diagnosis should evaluators use in child-custody litigation? *American Journal of Family Therapy, 30*(2), 93-115. https://doi.org/10.1080/019261802753573821

Godbout, É., & Parent, C. (2012). The life paths and lived experiences of adults who have experienced parental alienation: A retrospective study. *Journal of Divorce & Remarriage, 53*, 34-54. https://doi.org/10.1080/10502556.2012.635967

Gordon, R. M., Stoffey, R., & Bottinelli, J. (2008). MMPI-2 findings of primitive defenses in alienating patients. *American Journal of Family Therapy, 36*(3), 211–228. https://doi.org/10.1080/01926180701643313

Greenberg, J. R., & Mitchell, S. M. (1983). *Object relations in psychoanalytic theory*. Harvard University Press.

Greenberg, L. R., Fick, L. D., & Schnider, R. (2012). Keeping the developmental frame: Child-centered conjoint therapy. *Journal of Child Custody, 9*(1-2), 39–68. https://doi.org/10.1080/15379418.2012.652568

Greenberg, L. R., Fick, L. D., & Schnider, R. (2016). Catching them before too much damage is done: Early intervention with resistance-refusal dynamics. *Family Court Review, 54*(4), 548–563. https://doi.org/10.1111/fcre.12242

Greenberg, L., Fidler, B. J., & Saini, M. (Eds.). (2019). *Evidence-informed interventions for court-involved families*. Oxford University Press.

Gu, Y., Gu, S., Lei, Y., & Li, H. (2020). From uncertainty to anxiety: How uncertainty fuels anxiety in a process mediated by intolerance of uncertainty. *Neural Plasticity, 2020*. https://doi.org/10.1155/2020/8866386

Hamel, J., & Baker, K. (2022). Guidelines for domestic violence and child custody litigation. In B. Russel & J. Hamel (Eds.), *Gender and Domestic Violence: Contemporary Legal Practice and Intervention Reforms*. Oxford University Press.

Harman, J. J. & Matthewson, M. (2020). Parental Alienating Behaviors. In D. Lorandos & W. Bernet (Eds.), *Parental alienation: Science and law* (pp. 44-81). Charles C. Thomas, Publisher, Ltd.

Harman, J. J., & Lorandos, D. (2021). Allegations of family violence in court: How Parental Alienation affects judicial outcomes. *Psychology, Public Policy, and Law, 27*(2), 184–208. http://dx.doi.org/10.1037/law0000301

Harman, J. J., Kruk, E., & Hines, D. A. (2018). Parental alienating behaviors: an unacknowledged form of family violence. *Psychological Bulletin, 144*(12), 1275–1299. https://doi.org/10.1037/bul0000175

Harman, J. J., Saunders, L., & Afifi, T. (2021). Evaluation of the Turning Points for Families (TPFF) program for severely alienated children. *Journal of Family Therapy, 44*(2), 1-20. doi: 10.1111/1467-6427.12366

Harman, J. J., Warshak, R. A., Lorandos, D., & Florian, M. J. (2022). Developmental psychology and the scientific status of parental alienation. *Developmental Psychology, 58*(10), 1887-1911. https://doi.org/10.1037/dev0001404

Herman, S., & Freitas, T. R. (2010). Error rates in forensic child sexual abuse evaluations. *Psychological Injury and Law, 3*(2), 133-147. doi: 10.1007/s12207-010-9073-0

Herman, S. (2005). Improving decision making in forensic child sexual abuse evaluations. *Law and Human Behavior, 29*(1), 87-120. https://doi.org/10.1007/s10979-005-1400-8

Heyman, R. E., Slep, A. M. S., Eckardt Erlanger, A. C., & Foran, H. M. (2013). Intimate partner maltreatment: Definitions, prevalence, and implications for diagnosis. In H. M. Foran, S. R. H. Beach, A. M. S. Slep, R. E. Heyman, & M. Z. Wamboldt (Eds.), *Family problems and family violence: Reliable assessment and the ICD-11* (pp. 1-14). Springer Publishing Company.

Johnston, J. R., & Campbell, L. E. G. (1993). A clinical typology of interpersonal violence in disputed-custody cases. *American Journal of Orthopsychiatry, 63*(2), 190-199. doi:10.1037/h0079425

Johnston, J. R. (2005). Children of divorce who reject parent and refuse visitation: Recent research and social policy implications for the alienated child. *Family Law Quarterly, 38*(4), 757-776.

Johnston, J. R., & Campbell, L. E. G. (1988). *Impasses of divorce: The dynamics and resolution of family conflict.* Free Press.

Johnston, J. R., Campbell, L. E. G., & Mayes, S. S. (1985). Latency children in post-separation and divorce disputes. *Journal of the American Academy of Child Psychiatry, 24*(5), 563-574. https://doi.org/10.1016/s0002-7138(09)60057-1

Johnston, J. R., Lee, S., Olesen, N. W., & Walters, M. G. (2005). Allegations and substantiations of abuse in custody disputing families. *Family Court Review, 43*(2), 283-294. https://doi.org/10.1111/j.1744-1617.2005.00029.x

Johnston, J. R., & Roseby, V. (2009). Parental alignments and alienation among children of high-conflict divorce. In J. R. Johnston, V. Roseby, & K. Kuehnle (Eds.), *In the Name of the Child* (2nd ed., pp. 193-220). Simon and Schuster.

Johnston, J. R., Walters, M. G., & Friedlander, S. (2001). Therapeutic work with alienated children and their families. *Family Court Review, 39*(3), 316-333. https://doi.org/10.1111/j.174-1617.2001.tb00613.x

Johnston, J. R., Walters, M. G., & Olesen, N. W. (2005). Is It Alienating Parenting, Role Reversal or Child Abuse? A Study of Children's Rejection of a Parent in Child Custody Disputes. *Journal of Emotional Abuse, 5*(4), 191–218. https://doi.org/10.1300/J135v05n04_02

Judge, A. M., & Deutsch, R. M. (2017). *Overcoming parent-child contact problems: Family based interventions for resistance, rejection, and alienation.* Oxford University Press.

Kelly, J. B., & Johnston, J. R. (2001). The alienated child: A reformulation of parental alienation syndrome. *Family Court Review, 39*, 249-266. https://doi.org/10.1111/j.174-1617.2001.tb00609.x

Kendall-Tackett, K. A., Williams, L. M., & Finkelhor, D. (1993). Impact of sexual abuse on children: a review and synthesis of recent empirical studies. *Psychological Bulletin, 113*(1), 164-80. doi: 10.1037/0033-2909.113.1.164

Khalique, A., & Rohner, R. (2002). Perceived parent acceptance-rejection and psychological adjustment: A meta-analysis of cross-cultural and intracultural studies. *Journal of Marriage and the Family, 64*, 54–64. https://doi.org/10.1111/j.1741-3737.2002.00054.x

Klaff, R. L. (1982). The tender years doctrine: A defense. *California Law Review, 70*(2), 335- 372. https://doi.org/10.15779/Z38ZM97

Kovacs, M. (No year specified.). *Children's Depression Inventory 2nd Edition™ (CDI 2)* [Database record]. APA PsycTests. https://doi.org/10.1037/t04948-000

Kruk, E. (2018). Parental alienation as a form of emotional child abuse: The current state of knowledge and future directions for research. *Family Science Review*.

Kubler-Ross, E., & Kessler, E. (2014). *On grief and grieving.* Simon & Schuster.

Kuehnle, K., & Connell, M. (Eds.). (2009). *The evaluation of child sexual abuse allegations: A comprehensive guide to assessment and testimony.* John Wiley & Sons Inc.

Lampel, A. K. (1986). Post-divorce therapy with highly conflicted families. *Independent Practice, 6*(3), 22–26.

Levy, D. (1943). *Maternal Overprotection.* Norton & Company. urn: lcp:maternaloverprot0000levy:epub:426f9b07-0afb-41d3-8248-0aab60018a88

Lindahl, M. W. & Hunt, L. A. (2016). Reunification in intrafamilial child abuse cases: A model for intervention. *Family Court Review, 54*, 288-299. https://doi.org/10.1111/fcre.12219

Loftus, E. F. (1993). The reality of repressed memories. *American Psychologist, 48*(5), 518-537. https://doi.org/10.1037/0003-066X.48.5.518

Lorandos, D. (2020). Parental alienation in U.S. courts, 1985-2018. *Family Court Review, 58*(2), 322-339. https://doi.org/10.1111/fcre.12475

Lorandos, D., Bernet, W., & Sauber, S. R. (2013). Overview of parental alienation. In D. Lorandos, W. Bernet, S. R. Sauber, (Eds.), *Parental Alienation: The Handbook for Mental Health and Legal Professionals* (pp. 5-46). Charles C. Thomas, Publisher, Ltd.

MacKay, T. (2014). False allegations of child abuse in contested family law cases: The implications for psychological practice. *Educational and Child Psychology, 31*(3), 85-96. doi: 10.53841/bpsecp.2014.31.3.85

Main, M., Hesse, E., & Hesse, S. (2011). Attachment theory and research: Overview with suggested applications to child custody. *Family Court Review, 49,* 426–463.

Mason, M. A. (1994). *From father's property to children's rights: The history of child custody in the United States.* Columbia University Press.

McTavish, J. R., MacGregor, J. C. D., Wathen, C. N., & MacMillan, H. L. (2016). Children's exposure to intimate partner violence: an overview. *International Review of Psychiatry, 28*(5), 504–518. https://doi.org/10.1080/09540261.2016.1205001

Mercer, J., & Drew, M. (Eds.). (2021). *Challenging Parental Alienation: New Directions for Professionals and Parents* (1st ed.). Routledge. https://doi.org/10.4324/9781003095927

Minuchin, S. (1974). *Families and family therapy.* Harvard University Press.

Morrison, S. L. & Ring, R. (2021). Reliability of the Five-Factor Model for determining Parental Alienation. *The American Journal of Family Therapy, 51*(5), 580-598. https://doi.org/10.1080/01926187.2021.2021831

Myers, J. E. B. (2011). The short history of child protection in America. In J. E. B. Myers (Ed.), *The APSAC handbook on child maltreatment* (3rd ed.). Sage.

National Parents Organization, (2019). 2019 Shared parenting report card. National Parents Organization. Retrieved on August 20, 2024, from https://www.sharedparenting.org/2019- shared-parenting-report

Pearlin, L. I. (2010). The life course and the stress process: some conceptual comparisons. *The Journals of Gerontology. Series B, Psychological sciences and social sciences, 65B*(2), 207–215. https://doi.org/10.1093/geronb/gbp106

People ex rel. Watts v. Watts 77 Misc. 2d 178, 350 N.Y.S.2d 285 (1973).

Phifer, L., Crowder, A., Elsenraat, T., & Hull, R. (2017). *CBT Toolbox for Children and Adolescents: Over 200 Worksheets & Exercises for Trauma, ADHD, Autism, Anxiety, Depression & Conduct Disorders* (1st ed.). PESI Publishing & Media.

Polak, S. (2019). Mental Health Professionals' Practice of Reintegration Therapy for Parent–Child Contact Problems Post-separation: A Phenomenological Study. *Journal of Divorce & Remarriage, 61*(3), 225–248. https://doi.org/10.1080/10502556.2019.1699370

Polak, S. (2020). Mental health professionals' practice of reintegration therapy for parent–child contact problems post-separation: A phenomenological study. *Journal of Divorce & Remarriage, 61*(3), 225–248. https://doi.org/10.1080/10502556.2019.1699370

Polak, S., & Moran, J. A. (2017). The current status of outpatient approaches to parent–child contact problems. In A. M. Judge & R. M. Deutsch (Eds.), *Overcoming parent-child contact problems: Family-based interventions for resistance, rejection, and alienation* (pp. 63–90). Oxford Press.

Poole, D. A & Lindsay, D. S. (1998). Assessing the accuracy of young children's reports: Lessons from the investigation of child sexual abuse. *Journal of Applied and Preventive Psychology, 7*(1), 1-26. https://doi.org/10.1016/S0962-1849(98)80019-X

Professor Ross (2014, June 18). *Brain Games: False Memory and Misinformation Effect* [Video]. YouTube. https://www.youtube.com/watch?v=qQ-96BLaKYQ

Pruett, M. K., Arthur, L. A., & Ebling, R. (2007). The hand that rocks the cradle: Maternal gatekeeping after divorce. *Pace Law Review, 27*(4), 709-739. http://digitalcommons.pace.edu/plr/vol27/iss4/8

Rand, D. (1993). Munchausen Syndrome by Proxy: A complex type of emotional abuse responsible for some false allegations of child abuse in divorce. *IPT-Forensics Journal, 5*(3), 135-155. http://www.ipt-forensics.com/journal/volume5/j5_3_1.htm

Reay, K. M. (2015). Family reflections: A promising therapeutic program designed to treat severely alienated children and their family system. *The American Journal of Family Therapy, 43*, 197-207. doi: 10.1080/01926187.2015.1007769

Reich, W. (1949). *Character-analysis* (3rd ed.). Orgone Institute Press.

Rex v. de Manneville, 102 Eng. Rep. 1054 (1804). The King against De Manneville - Case Law - VLEX 803373289

Reynolds, C. R., & Richmond, B. O. (2008). *Reynolds Child Manifest Anxiety Scale, Second Edition (RCMAS-2)*. Western Psychological Services.

Rohner, R. P. (2005). *Parental Acceptance-Rejection Questionnaire (PARQ): Test manual*. In R. P. Rohner & A. Khaleque (Eds.), *Handbook for the study of parental acceptance and rejection* (4th ed., pp. 43-106). Rohner Research Publications.

Roma, P., Marchetti, D., Mazza, C., Ricci, E., Fontanesi, L., & Verrocchio, M. C. (2022). A Comparison of MMPI-2 Profiles Between Parental Alienation Cases and Custody Cases. *Journal of Child and Family Studies, 31*, 1196–1206. https://doi.org/10.1007/s10826-021-02076-1

Rosenberg, M. (1965). *Society and the adolescent self-image*. Princeton University Press.

Rowen, J. & Emery, R. (2014). Examining parental denigration behaviors of coparents as reported by young adults and their associations with parent-child closeness. *Couples and Family Psychology: Research and Practice, 3*(3), 165-177. https://doi.org/10.1037/cfp0000026

Rowen, J. & Emery, R. (2018). Parental denigration: A form of conflict that generally backfires. *Family Court Review, 56*(2), 258-268. https://doi.org/10.1111/fcre.12339

Ryan Thomas Speaks. (2015). They ambushed my dad: Child of Parental Alienation. [Video]. YouTube. https://www.youtube.com/watch?v=jzV1cRw7_MQ

Saini, M., Johnston, J. R., Fidler, B. J., & Bala, N. (2016). Empirical studies of alienation. In L. Drozd, M. Saini, & N. Olesen (Eds.), *Parenting plan evaluations: Applied research for the family court* (2nd ed., pp. 374–430). Oxford University Press. https://doi.org/10.1093/med:psych/9780199396580.003.0013

Saini, M., Laajasalo, T., & Platt, S. (2020). Gatekeeping by allegations: An examination of verified, unfounded, and fabricated allegations of child maltreatment within the context of resist and refusal dynamics. *Family Court Review, 58*(2), 417–431. https://doi.org/10.1111/fcre.12480

Saunders, D. G., & Faller, K. C. (2016). The need to carefully screen for family violence when parental alienation is claimed. *Michigan Family Law Journal, 46*(6), 7–11.

Saunders, M. R., Morawska, A., Haslam, D. M., & Fletcher, R. (2014). Parenting and family adjustment scales (PAFAS): Validation of a brief parent-report measure for use in assessment of parenting skills and family relationships. *Child Psychiatry & Human Development, 5*(3), 255-272. https://eprints.qut.edu.au/220784/

Schneider, P. (Director). (1995). *Indictment: The McMartin Trial* [Film]. CBS Productions.

Shaw, J. (2016, February 17). *Julia Shaw on "Memory Hackers" NOVA* [Video]. YouTube. https://www.youtube.com/watch?v=NfPLTtlo2oY

Silberg, J., & Dallam, S. (2019). Abusers gaining custody in family courts: A case series of overturned decisions. *Journal of Child Custody, 16*(2), 140–169. https://doi.org/10.1080/15379418.2019.1613204

Smith, L. (2016). Family-based therapy for parent–child reunification. *Journal of Clinical Psychology: In Session, 72*(5), 498–512. https://doi.org/10.1002/jclp.22259

Sullivan, M. (2019). Building and managing collaborative teams. In L. R. Greenberg, B. J. Fidler, & M. A. Saini (Eds.), *Evidence-Informed Interventions for Court Involved Families* (pp. 355-374). Oxford University Press.

Teichman, J. (1982). *Illegitimacy: A philosophical examination.* Basil Blackwell Publisher Limited.

Templer, K., Matthewson, M., Haines, J., & Cox, G. (2017). Recommendations for best practice in response to parental alienation: findings from a systematic review. *Journal of Family Therapy, 39*(1), 103-122. https://doi.org/10.1111/1467-6427.12137

The Supreme Court's Parental Rights Doctrine (n.d.). Parental Rights. Retrieved August 20, 2024, from https://parentalrights.org/understand_the_issue/supreme-court/

Trocmé, N. & Bala, N. (2005). False allegations of abuse and neglect when parents separate. *Child Abuse & Neglect, 29*(12), 1333-1345. https://doi.org/10.1016/j.chiabu.2004.06.016

Verrocchio, M. C., Marchetti, D., Roma, P., & Ferracuti, S. (2018). Relational and psychological features of high-conflict couples who engage in parental alienation. *Ricerche di Psicologia, 41*(4), 679–692. https://doi.org/10.3280/RIP2018-004008

Wallerstein J. S., & Kelly J. B. (1976). The effects of parental divorce: experiences of the child in later latency. *American Journal of Orthopsychiatry. 46*(2), 256-269. DOI: 10.1111/j.1939-0025.1976.tb00926.x

Walters, M. G., & Friedlander, S. (2010). Finding a tenable middle space: Understanding the role of clinical interventions when a child refuses contact with a parent. *Journal of Child Custody: Research, Issues, and Practices, 7*(4), 287- 328. https://doi.org/10.1080/15379418.2010.521027

Walters, M. G., & Friedlander, S. (2010). Finding a Tenable Middle Space: Understanding the Role of Clinical Interventions When a Child Refuses Contact with a Parent. *Journal of Child Custody, 7*(4), 287–328. https://doi.org/10.1080/15379418.2010.521027

Walters, M. G., & Friedlander, S. (2016). When a child rejects a parent: Working with the intractable resist/refuse dynamic. *Family Court Review, 54*(3), 424-445. https://doi.org/10.1111/fcre.12238

Warshak, R. A. (2010). Family Bridges: Using insights from social science to reconnect parents and alienated children. *Family Court Review 48(1),* 48-80. http://dx.doi.org/10.1111/j.1744-1617.2009.01288.x

Warshak, R. A. (2013). Severe cases of Parental Alienation. In D. Lorandos, W. Bernet, & S. R. Sauber (Eds.), *Parental Alienation: The Handbook for Mental Health and Legal Professionals* (pp. 125-162). Charles C. Thomas, Publisher, Ltd.

Warshak, R. A. (2015). Parental alienation: Overview, management, intervention and practice tips. *Journal of the American Academy of Matrimonial Lawyers, 28*: 181-248.

Warshak, R. A. (2015). The ten parental alienation fallacies that compromise decisions in court and in therapy. *Professional Psychology: Research and Practice, 46*(4), 235–249.

Warshak, R. A. (2018). Reclaiming parent-child relationships. Outcomes of Family Bridges with Alienated Children, of *Journal Divorce & Remarriage, 60*(8), 645-667. https://doi.org/10.1080/10502556.2018.1529505

Warshak, R. A. (2020). Parental alienation: How to prevent, manage, and remedy it. In D. Lorandos & W. Bernet (Eds.), *Parental Alienation: Science and Law* (pp. 142-206). Charles C. Thomas, Publisher, Ltd.

Warshak, R. A. (2020). Risks and realities of working with alienated children. *Family Court Review, 58*(2), 432-455. https://doi.org/10.1111/fcre.12481

Wheaton, M. G., Messner, G. R., & Marks, J. B. (2021). Intolerance of uncertainty as a factor linking obsessive-compulsive symptoms, health anxiety and concerns about the spread of the novel coronavirus (COVID-19) in the United States. *Journal of Obsessive-Compulsive and Related Disorders, 28,* 100605. Doi.org/10.1016/j.jocrd.2020.100605.

Woodall, K. (2017, June 21). Hurting the heart of a child: Parental alienation is child abuse. *Karen Woodall Blog.* https://karenwoodall.blog/2017/06/21/hurting-the-heart-of-a-child-parental-alienation-is-child-abuse/

Woodall, K. & Woodall, N. (2017). *Understanding Parental Alienation: Learning to Cope, Helping to Heal.* Charles C. Thomas, Publisher, Ltd.

Worenklein, A. (2013). Moderate cases of parental alienation. In D. Lorandos, W. Bernet, & R. Sauber (Eds.), *Parental alienation: The handbook for mental health and legal professionals* (pp. 97-124). Charles C. Thomas, Publisher, Ltd.

Zunshine, L. (2005). *Bastards and foundlings: Illegitimacy in eighteenth-century England.* Ohio State University Press.

SUBJECT INDEX

A

Abduction reunification, 192
Abuse. *See* Child abuse
Abuse allegations: differentiating between estrangement and parental alienation
   abused children compared to alienated, 61–63, 63*f*
   alienating behavior strategies, 29–30, 65–67, 139–140
   ambiguity of allegations, 52–53
   characteristics unique to alienated children, 79, 89, 145, 159, 190–191
   Conceptual Framework Hypothesis, 55
   estrangement, 30–31, 75, 77*f*
   factors to assess, 54, 57, 92, 209
   five-factor model of parental alienation, 57–70
   intervention with a targeted parent, 143, 152
   interviewer flaws, 56
   MHP guidelines, 56
   reporting abuse allegations, 78
   research findings on, 54–55, 57
Affidavits, 216–218
Age as a factor in children, 23–24. *See also* Developmental factors
Alignments. *See* Family dynamics in parent-child contact issues
A Little Spot of Emotion (Alber), 119
"All About Me" games and activities, 108, 118

Ambiguity, 165
Ambiguous loss, 142–143, 157–169. *See also* Grief and loss
Ambivalence, 164–165
American Professional Society on the Abuse of Children (APSAC), 14
Anxiety
   about treatment, 173, 183
   Beck Anxiety Inventory (BAI), 39
   children predisposed to, 26
   coping strategies children use, 73–74
   in enmeshment, 27
   expressed by alienated children, 90–91, 152
   in favored parents, 135
   as a focus in treatment, 174
   Reynolds Children's Manifest Anxiety Scale—2nd Edition, 124
   in targeted parents, 152, 156–157, 165, 174
   during transitions, 41–42, 99–100, 146
Apps for tracking emotions, 119, 123–124
Assessment procedures for mental health clinicians
   areas of investigation for causes of resistance, 48–49, 76
   case vignettes, 44–46
   child as client, 42–43
   Clinician's Toolbox, 49–51, 124
   collateral contacts, 37–38, 92
   differentiating estrangement and alienation, 77*f*, 92

differentiating resistance or refusal, 42
family dynamics, 34–35
family of origin information, 40–41
grief and loss evaluation, 156
historical timelines, 40, 60
legal information, 35–37
neutrality/bias, 46–48
parents as clients, 43–44
reactions to intervention, 44–46
studies on assessment models for parental alienation, 10
testing instruments, 38–40, 124
transitions and exchanges, 41–42
Association of Family and Conciliation Courts (AFCC), 56, 208, 211–215, 221
Attachment, 22–23, 62, 64–65, 129, 165–166

B

Beck Anxiety Inventory (BAI), 39
Beck Depression Inventory (BDI-II), 39
Best interest standard, 5–6
"Beyond the high road: Responding to 17 strategies of parental alienation without compromising your morals or harming your child," 148, 152
Bibliotherapy for children, 110–112, 115, 119
BIFF approach at communication, 134–135, 139
BIFF for Coparent Communication: Your Guide to Difficult Texts, Emails, and Social Media Posts (Eddy), 176
Black-and-white thinking. *See under* Cognitive distortions
Blogs, 171
Boundaries
developmental perspective on, 95, 109
with favored parents, 27
between households, 108–109, 134, 176–180
in therapy, 93, 173
Bowen, Murray, 7, 73–74
Buckey; People v. (1983), 54

C

Causes of parent-child contact issues
attachment, 22–23
case vignettes, 19–20, 24, 32
child characteristics in, 23–26, 50
family dynamics with unhealthy alignments, 26–33, 98–99
historical look at, 3, 6–8, 76
intimate partner/domestic violence, 18–19
loyalty conflicts, 16–17
parental conflict pre- and post-separation, 18–20
parent characteristics, 20–22
reactions to circumstances of divorce, 17–18
CBT Toolbox for Children and Adolescents, 123
Center for Missing and Exploited Children, 192
Child abuse. *See also* Abuse allegations: differentiating between estrangement and parental alienation
bonding to the abuser, 62
Munchausen Syndrome by Proxy (MSP), 11
psychological, 13–14, 63–64, 75, 206
sexual abuse allegations, 11, 53–55
"Child Affected by Parental Relationship Distress (CAPRD)," 13, 72–74
Children Held Hostage (Clawar and Rivlin), 10–11
Child's best interest, 3–5
Child support, 3–4
Child treatment
case vignettes, 105–106, 116–117

Clinician's Toolbox, 123
establishing the degree of resistance, 102–103, 173
finding authentic experience, 102, 104
issues to consider, 97–98
lifting the burden, 99–101
in Multi-Modal Family Intervention (MMFI), 199
providing protected psychological space, 101–106
psychological instruments, 121–122
recommendations when progress stalls, 122

Child treatment goals
Goal #1–Build Rapport, 103–106
Goal #2–Build Self-Esteem, 106–108
Goal #3–Help Child Individuate from Both Parents, 108–112
Goal #4–Develop Critical Thinking Skills, 112–117
Goal #5–Integrate Psychological Split, 117–118
Goal #6–Decrease Anxiety and Trauma Responses, 118–120
Goal #7–Decrease Shame and Guilt, 120–121

Child treatment techniques
addressing distortions, 113–114, 117–118
bibliotherapy and games, 110–112, 119, 123
building a covert therapeutic alliance, 105
Calming Bottle or Sensory Bottle, 120
Coping Bag, 119–120
developing coping strategies, 118
empathy, 104–105, 114
psychoeducation, 109, 114–115, 120–121
therapeutic activities, 108
when progress stalls, 122

Cognitive dissonance, 17

Cognitive distortions
black-and-white thinking, 112–113, 117, 130
clinical perspective on, 13
splitting, 136, 149, 199
techniques for addressing, 113–117, 130–131, 187
treatment planning for, 89, 93, 96, 103

Collective support, 26
Communication, 65, 134–135, 139, 174, 176
Confirmation bias, 47–48
Consequences of rejecting a parent, 25, 99, 129, 161
Context of children's problems, 74–75
Continuing education, 207–208
Coping Bag, 119–120
Coping mechanisms, 25, 178. *See also* Defense mechanisms
Coping with Cross-Examination and other Pathways to Effective Testimony (Brodsky), 221
Counter-productive protective parenting, 12

Court Orders. *See also* Formalized treatment agreements
court-ordered therapy, 83–84, 210–213
parental compliance with, 127–128, 175
for reunification treatment, 191, 197, 199–201
in treatment planning, 80–82, 172–173
types of, 210–211

Cross-generational coalitions, 7–8

Custody evaluations
availability of, 35
as a collateral resource, 70
PARQ used in, 38
role of, 217
scope of, 37, 202, 213
terminology used by, 14

D

Defense mechanisms, 20–21, 135–136,

149, 164. *See also* Coping mechanisms
de Manneville v. de Manneville (1804): early custody case, 4
Dependency cultivation, 28, 67
Depositions, 216
Depression
  Beck Depression Inventory (BDI-II), 39
  case vignette illustrating, 155–156
  children predisposed to, 26
  Children's Depression Inventory, 124
  in favored parents, 135
  in targeted parents, 22, 156, 163, 165
Developmental factors
  age related preferences, 23–24, 49
  assessment of, 49–51, 90, 110
  caretakers in early childhood, 5–6
  developmentally appropriate parenting, 148–149
  impediments to healthy development, 28, 67, 99, 109, 179
  in parenting roles, 148–149, 156
Diagnostic considerations
  "Child Affected by Parental Relationship Distress (CAPRD)," 13, 72–76
  differences and similarities between alienation and estrangement, 77f
  interpersonal violence and distress, 75–76
  levels of resistance and alienating behaviors, 77–79, 79f, 173
  parental alienation, 76–77
  parental behaviors that cause rejection of a parent, 78–79
  parent-child relational problem (PCRP) and child psychological abuse, 74–75
Dialectical thinking, 163–164, 171
Disillusionment, 160
Divorce
  child protective agencies involved in, 60
  historical overview of, 4–6
  issues in high conflict situations, 6, 72, 98, 106–107
  trauma of litigation, 166
Documentation/evidence, 29, 77, 82, 85–86, 89
Domestic violence, 18–19, 72, 75–76
DSM-5 (APA, 2013), 63–64, 71–72, 74–76

E

Education. *See* Psychoeducation of parents
Educational information, 151–152, 163–164
Emotional dysregulation, 21
Emotions Uno (game), 119, 123
Empathy, 158
Empowerment, 150–151, 153–154, 156, 179
Enmeshment, 27–28, 50, 98, 109–110
Estrangement, 30–31, 75, 77f. *See also* Abuse allegations: differentiating between estrangement and parental alienation
The Expert Expert Witness: More Maxims and Guidelines for Testifying in Court (Brodsky), 221
Extracurricular activities impacting therapy scheduling, 85–86, 95, 176, 178

F

False accusations, 19, 206
False memories and suggestibility, 133, 139
Families in Transition (program), 38
Family Bridges Aftercare Protocol, 136
Family Bridges program, 191–195
Family dynamics in parent-child contact issues
  evaluating, 15–16, 34–35
  literature review of, 6–8
  parental resistance, 85

power dynamics, 40
treatment goals for, 93
unhealthy alignments, 26–33
Family of origin issues, 33, 40–41, 127–129
The Family Reflections Reunification Program, 208–210
Family treatment
case vignettes, 181, 188
Clinician's Toolbox, 189
considerations with siblings, 187–188
context for, 172–174
goals and techniques for working with parents, 175–178
Parent and Family Member Pledge to Child, 177–178
recommendations when progress stalls, 188–189
responding to accusations, 184
therapeutic foci of treatment, 174–175
working with the favored parent-child dyad, 178–181
working with the target parent-child dyad, 182–188
Favored parent treatment
Goal #1—Follow the Court Order, 127
Goal #2—Understand Their Own Family of Origin Dynamics, 127–129
Goal #3—Support the Relationship Between the Child and the Targeted Parent, 128–130
Goal #4—Increase Insight and Take Responsibility, 130–131
Goal #5—Increase Ability to Cooperatively Parallel Parent, 133–135
case vignettes, 127–128, 138–139
Clinician's Toolbox, 139–140
mental health issues interfering with, 135–137
parental alienation strategies, 131–132, 139–140
recommendations for stalled progress, 137–139
suggestibility and false memories, 133
therapeutic foci of treatment, 125–126
working with the favored parent-child dyad, 178–181
Fees related to providing testimony, 219
Fiona the Flamingo (Chu and Jeffery), 119
Five Love Languages (Chapman), 144–145
"Folie a' deux" relationships, 11
Forensic evaluations
accessing, 35, 49
appropriate interviewing in, 53
case example, 46
decision making model for, 12
psychological tests used in, 37
scope of, 13
used to differentiate causes of contact refusal, 76
Formalized treatment agreements, 94–96. *See also* Court Orders
Fourteenth Amendment, 5
Frankl, Victor, 158, 160
Freud, Sigmund, 164

G

Games for use with children in therapy, 108, 111–112, 115–116, 119
Gardner, Richard, 8–10, 14, 60, 67, 112
Grief and loss, 156–157, 166. *See also* Ambiguous loss

H

"The hand that rocks the cradle: Maternal gatekeeping after divorce," 12–13. *See also Maternal Overprotection* (Levy)
Health information, 151–152
HIPAA, 37
History of child custody, 3–6
Hope as a therapeutic focus, 150–156, 158, 161, 166–168

I

Identity reconstruction, 162–164
"Indictment: The McMartin Trial" (movie), 54
Infantilization, 28, 67
In My Body, I Feel (Flynn), 119
Intake process during treatment planning, 83
The International Council on Shared Parenting (ICSP), 208
Intervention informing assessment, 44–46, 88
Intimate partner distress (IPD), 72, 75
Intimate partner violence, 18–19, 72, 75–76

J

The Journal of American Academy of Child & Adolescent Psychiatry, 72
Justice, 161–163

K

Kubler-Ross, E., 166

L

Legal information as an assessment resource, 35–37
Legal orders. *See* Court orders
Listening to My Body (Garcia), 119
Literature on parental alienation, 207–208
"The Little Boy and the Beast" (video), 105, 123
Loyalty binds or conflicts
   assessing for, 76
   in *DSM-5*, 13
   dynamics of, 16–17, 53, 73–74
   educating parents about, 145
   including in agreements, 95
   protected psychological space alleviating, 101–102
   research about, 8
Ludmer, Brian, 95–96

M

Man's Search for Meaning (Frankl), 158
Margaret Kelly Michaels v. New Jersey (1985), 54
Mastery, tempering of, 160–162
Maternal Overprotection (Levy), 6–7. *See also* The hand that rocks the cradle: Maternal gatekeeping after divorce
Meaning, search for, 158–160, 166
"Memory Hackers" (documentary), 115, 123, 139
Mental health issues, 135–137, 157, 161, 209. *See also specific disorders*
Minuchin, Salvador, 7, 73–74, 194
Multi-Modal Family Intervention (MMFI), 199
Munchausen Syndrome by Proxy (MSP), 11
Music used in therapy, 112

O

Optimism, 162

P

Parallel parenting plans, 135
Parental Acceptance and Rejection Questionnaire (PARQ), 38–39, 121–122, 190
Parental alienation; five-factor model of
   overview of, 57–58
   Factor One-resistance, 58–59, 173
   Factor Two-prior positive relationship, 59–60
   Factor Three-absence of abuse, 60–63
   Factor Four-alienating behaviors of favored parent, 63–67
   Factor Five-child characteristics, 67–70

Subject Index

Parental Alienation (PA)
    assessing, 50–51, 54, 57
    characteristics unique to alienated children, 79, 89, 145, 159, 190–191
    dynamics of, 28–30
    hybrid cases of PA with estrangement, 31–32
    literature review on, 6–8
    parental alienation strategies, 131–132
    Parental Alienation Syndrome (PAS), 8–14
    pathological alienation, 12
    "reformulation" of parental alienation (PA), 11–12
    terminology update to, 10
    "The Ten Parental Alienation Fallacies that Compromise Decisions in Court and in Therapy," 89–90
Parental Alienation Study Group (PASG), 158, 208
The Parental Alienation Syndrome (Gardner), 9–10, 14
Parental Rights Doctrine, Supreme Court's, 3
Parent and Family Member Pledge to Child, 177–178
Parentification, 28
Parenting skills, 147
Parenting Stress Index (PSI), 39–40
Personality and projective testing, 37
Personality disorders, 135–136, 209
Pessimism, 162
Professional liability and protecting yourself
    areas of concern, 205–206
    assessing treatment effectiveness, 214–215
    Clinician's Toolbox, 221
    continuing education, 207–208
    court-ordered therapy, 210–213
    professional role boundaries, 36, 213, 217, 220
    review treatment progress, 208–210
    risks of working with alienated children, 206, 214
    social media, 207
    testifying in court, 215–221
Psychoeducation of parents
    about loyalty binds, 17, 64, 145, 174
    on benefits of parental relationships, 129
    on developmental phases, 148–149
    on diffusing conflict, 170
    in Family Bridges program, 192
    on impact of alienating behaviors, 77–78
    regarding communication, 134–135
    on suggestibility and false memories, 133
    topics for targeted parents, 141–142
    in Turning Points for Families (TPFF), 194

R

Resilience/vulnerability, 25, 139, 160–164
"Resist-refusal" dynamics
    assessing, 43, 48–49, 76
    complexity of, 98–99
    developers of model for, 13
    documentation of, 77
    forms of resistance, 83–84
    in hybrid cases, 22
    levels of resistance and alienating behaviors, 58–59, 77–79, 79*f*, 173
Reunification
    barriers during process of, 185
    expectations about the process, 176, 179, 210
    programs, 159
    sabotage of, 178
    treatment, 61–62, 95, 173
Rigidity, 21

S

Sabotage of therapy, 81, 84–85, 88–89
Safety plans for initial child(ren) visits, 169–170
Secrets, 160, 179
Self-care, 154
Self-esteem, 25, 106–108, 124
Seligman, Martin, 162
Sexual abuse allegations, 11
Siblings, 187–188
Six Thinking Hats (game), 115–116, 123
Social media, 206–207
Special needs children, 23
Splitting. *See under* Cognitive distortions
Stigma of rejection, 157–158
Stubbornness, 25
Subpoenas, 215
Substance abuse, 30–33
Suggestibility and false memories, 133
Support groups for parents of alienated children, 167, 171
Supreme Court Parental Rights Doctrine, 3
Symbolic Communications, 65
Systems-level perspective, 42–43

T

Targeted parent treatment
    Goal #1 – Build Rapport and Trust, 142–145
    Goal #2—Shift from Anger and Betrayal to Empathy and Compassion, 145–146
    Goal #3—Improve Parenting Skills, 147–150
    Goal #4—Increase Feelings of Hope and Empowerment, 150–155
    Goal #5—Coping with Grief and Loss, 156–167
    Goal #6—Preparing the Parent for Therapeutic Contact with the Child, 168–169
    Goal #7—Preparing the Parent to Receive the Child in Their Home, 169–170
    ambiguous loss, 157–158
    case vignettes, 150–151, 153–156
    Clinician's Toolbox, 171
    developmentally appropriate parenting, 148–149
    getting to know the child, 144–145
    parenting alienated children, 147–148
    processing ambiguous losses, 158–169
    responses to accusations, 184
    restoring authority, 183
    reunification preparation, 149
    tempering mastery, 160–162
    therapeutic foci of treatment, 141–142
    working with the target parent-child dyad, 182–188
Tender Years' Doctrine, 5
Terminology for parent-child contact issues, 14
Testifying in court, 215–221
Testing instruments, 38–40, 121–122
Texas Children's Bill of Rights, 177, 179
"Third-party alienation," 208–209
"Tiger-Tiger, Is It True?" (Katie & Wilhelm), 115
Transgenerational haunting, 33, 127
"Transition bridge," 41, 99–100, 146
Trauma, 33
Treatment of parent-child contact issues. *See also* Psychoeducation of parents
    barriers to treatment success, 94
    collaboration used in, 94, 103, 200
    determining route to resistance, 16, 64
Treatment planning
    assessment, 90–93
    child's resistance to therapy, 88–89
    court-involved clients, 80–82
    extracurricular activities, 86
    formalized treatment agreements, 94–96
    forms of resistance, 83–84, 88, 94

goals of treatment planning, 89, 92
intake process, 83
intrusiveness, 87–88
legal orders, 82
research findings on rejection, 91
scheduling issues, 84–86
stalling the start of therapy, 86–87
treatment goals, 93–94
vignette, 88
why traditional therapy might not work, 89–91
Treatment team models of intervention for severe cases of parental alienation
    Clinician's Toolbox, 204
    Family Bridges program, 191–194
    Family Reflections Reunification Program (FRRP), 195–197
    overview of, 190–191
    therapeutic treatment teams, 197–204
Turning Points for Families (TPFF), 194–195
Triangulation dynamic, 26–27, 73–74
Turning Points for Families (TPFF), 194–195

V

Vulnerability/resilience in children, 25

W

Weaponization of children, 14
Wee Care childcare case, 56
"What Parents Need to Know from Kids About Divorce" (video), 104–105, 123
Workbooks for children, 110
Worksheets and resources addressing cognitive distortions, 114
Would you rather (game), 111–112, 123

CHARLES C THOMAS • PUBLISHER • LTD.

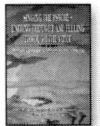

SINGING THE PSYCHE—UNITING THOUGHT AND FEELING THROUGH THE VOICE
Anne M. Brownell, Deirdre A. Brownell and Gina Holloway Mulder
320 pp. (7 x 10) • 22 illustrations
$28.95 (paper) • $28.95 (ebook)

TRAUMA INFORMED DRAMA THERAPY
Nisha Sajnani and David Read Johnson
350 pp. (7 x 10) • 8 illustrations
$49.95 (paper) • $49.95 (ebook)

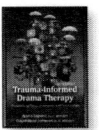

DEVELOPING ISSUES IN WORLD MUSIC THERAPY
Karen D. Goodman
368 pp. (7 x 10) • 8 illustrations • 9 tables
$56.95 (paper) • $56.95 (ebook)

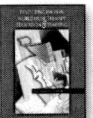

ATTUNEMENT IN EXPRESSIVE ARTS THERAPY
(2nd Ed.)
Mitchell Kossak
234 pp. (7 x 10) • 28 illustrations
$38.95 (paper) • $38.95 (ebook)

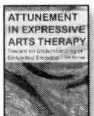

THERAPEUTIC ALLIANCE IN INTEGRATIVE ADDICTIONS-FOCUSED PSYCHOTHERAPY AND COUNSELING
Gary G. Forrest
376 pp. (7 x 10) • 1 table
$60.95 (paper) • $60.95 (ebook)

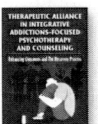

HELPING STUDENTS WITH DISABILITIES DEVELOP SOCIAL SKILLS, ACADEMIC LANGUAGE AND LITERACY THROUGH LITERATURE STORIES, VIGNETTES, AND OTHER ACTIVITIES
Elva Duran
608 pp. (7 x 10) • 26 illustrations • 4 tables
$54.95 (comb) • $54.95 (ebook)

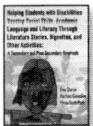

THE HANDBOOK OF CHILD LIFE
(2nd Ed.)
Richard H. Thompson
642 pp. (7 x 10) • 7 illustrations • 14 tables
$65.95 (paper) • $65.95 (ebook)

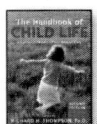

WHEN PARENTS HAVE PROBLEMS
(3rd Ed.)
Susan B. Miller
130 pp. (7 x 10)
$21.95 (paper) • $21.95 (ebook)

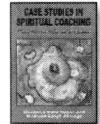

CASE STUDIES IN SPIRITUAL COACHING
DeeAnna Merz Nagel and Madison Leigh Akridge
276 pp. (7 x 10) • 6 illustrations
$41.95 (paper) • $41.95 (ebook)

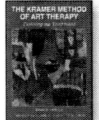

THE KRAMER METHOD OF ART THERAPY
David R. Henley
252 pp. (7 x 10) • 94 illustrations (8 in color)
$39.95 (paper) • $39.95 (ebook)

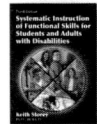

SYSTEMATIC INSTRUCTION OF FUNCTIONAL SKILLS FOR STUDENTS AND ADULTS WITH DISABILITIES
(3rd Ed.)
Keith Storey
292 pp. (7 x 10) • 14 illustrations • 35 tables
$48.95 (paper) • $48.95 (ebook)

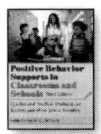

POSITIVE BEHAVIOR SUPPORTS IN CLASSROOMS AND SCHOOLS (3rd Ed.)
Keith Storey
300 pp. (7 x 10) • 15 illustrations • 53 tables
$46.95 (paper) • $46.95 (ebook)

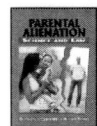

PARENTAL ALIENATION— SCIENCE AND LAW
Demosthenes Lorandos and William Bernet
682 pp. (7 x 10) • 4 illustrations • 12 tables
$74.95 (hard) • $74.95 (ebook)

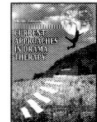

CURRENT APPROACHES IN DRAMA THERAPY
(3rd Ed.)
David Read Johnson and Renée Emunah
624 pp. (7 x 10) • 5 illustrations
$95.95 (paper) • $95.95 (ebook)

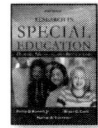

RESEARCH IN SPECIAL EDUCATION
(3rd Ed.)
Phillip D. Rumrill, Jr., Bryan G. Cook and Nathan A. Stevenson
300 pp. (7 x 10) • 3 illustrations • 4 tables
$49.95 (paper) • $49.95 (ebook)

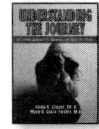

UNDERSTANDING THE JOURNEY
Hilda R. Glazer and Myra Clark-Foster
272 pp. (7 x 10) • 13 illustrations • 3 tables
$43.95 (paper) • $43.95 (ebook)

FREE SHIPPING ON RETAIL PURCHASES NOW AVAILABLE!*

Find us on: facebook.
FACEBOOK.COM/CCTPUBLISHER

*Available on retail purchases through our website only to domestic shipping addresses in the United States

TO ORDER: www.ccthomas.com • 1-800-258-8980 • books@ccthomas.com
Go to www.ccthomas.com and sign up for our e-Newsletter for New Releases. Be the first to know!